The Call to
WHOLENESS

The Call to
WHOLENESS

HEALTH AS A
SPIRITUAL JOURNEY

Kenneth L. Bakken

CROSSROAD • NEW YORK

1992

The Crossroad Publishing Company
370 Lexington Avenue, New York, N.Y. 10017

Library of Congress Cataloging in Publication Data
Bakken, Kenneth L.
    The call to wholeness.
    Bibliography: p. 114
    1. Health—Religious aspects—Christianity.
    2. Christian life—1960-   I. Title. II. Title:
Health as a spiritual journey.
BT732.B335 1985   248.4   84-23837
ISBN 0-8245-0683-9 (pbk.)

Grateful acknowledgment is made for permission to quote from the following books:
    The Call to Conversion by Jim Wallis. Copyright © 1981 by Sojourners. Reprinted by
permission of Harper and Row, Publishers, Inc.
    Encounter with God by Morton Kelsey. Published and copyright 1972, Bethany House
Publishers, Minneapolis, MN 55438. Reprinted by permission.
    The Other Side of Silence by Morton T. Kelsey. Copyright © 1976 by The Missionary
Society of St. Paul the Apostle in the State of New York. Reprinted by permission of
Paulist Press.
    The Turning Point by Fritjof Capra. Copyright © 1981 by Fritjof Capra. Reprinted by
permission of Simon & Schuster, Inc.

Unless otherwise indicated, all scriptural quotations are from the Revised Standard
Version of the Bible.

Contents

To Mom and Dad

Foreword

There is no question that Jesus was interested in healing the souls, bodies, and minds of the people who were oppressed by sickness, darkness, and pain. These people flocked around him to listen to his words and to be healed by his touch or even as they touched the hem of his garment. Jesus did not require anything of those who came for healing except that they be open to receive his healing power. In the same way when Jesus rose from the dead and so defeated the forces of evil, he did it not only for the good or the repentent but for all men and women, good and bad, if only they would turn and receive his grace. One of the church fathers wrote that the gift of healing in the church was indeed the first fruit, the first consequence, of the resurrection.

Any honest reading of the four gospels shows that a major portion of Jesus' ministry was spent in healing the sick. Nearly a fifth of the total verses of the gospels describes these healings. As the church grew we find the spirit of Jesus, the Holy Spirit, operating in the church. We find the same practice of healing among the apostles recorded in the book of Acts. One of the most significant characteristics of the early church—when the Christian community was at its finest and strongest—was the healing ministry. The pagans sneered at Christians because sick and sinful people were acceptable to their God. The emperor Julian, who tried to ban Christianity and to make paganism the religion of the Roman Empire in the late fourth century, wrote: "Now we can see what makes Christians such powerful enemies of our gods. It is the brotherly love which they manifest toward strangers and toward the sick and the poor." In *Healing and Christianity* I described how the ministry of sacramental healing continued in the life of the church until the spirit of secular materialism invaded most of our institutions, even the church, in the past two hundred years.

In Jesus' time the medical profession did not offer much in the way of healing. I am certain that had Jesus lived in our day he would have used medical means of healing as well as sacramental-spiritual means. Jesus was a very practical person. The first free hospitals and hospices to care for the sick and the dying were built by Christians. Mother Teresa of Calcutta is carrying on the tradition of the early church. Even when the church no longer believed that it had any power to help and transform the whole human being through religious or sacramental methods, it still built hospitals and cared for the destitute. God created the whole world and gave us the potential for both medical, psychological, and spiritual-sacramental healing. We are using only a portion of God's gifts if we do not use all three of the means of renewal and transformation. And still there are very few places in the Christian church where all three of these valid ways of healing are used together.

The finest attempt to bring these aspects of healing together that I know of is St. Luke Health Ministries in Baltimore, Maryland. Here doctors and nurses with a profound understanding of the church's spiritual-sacramental ministry work with men and women with psychological and religious training to provide care for the whole person, both mind and soul. It is easy to have ideas about this kind of care; it is quite another thing to provide such care.

The Call to Wholeness is written by one of the physicians involved in St. Luke Health Ministries and one of its founders. Dr. Kenneth Bakken not only describes the theory behind their work but also speaks out of several years of working in this environment. He also teaches at the Johns Hopkins University School of Public Health. This book presents sickness in terms of injury to the whole person. Obviously real healing and wholeness can only come when the whole person is involved. Fear is perceived as the destroyer that attacks all of us. Love is understood as the reality that can begin to deliver us from fear and lead us to the source of love, the resurrected Christ who has conquered evil and fear. Seeking for health can be a pathway to wholeness and an invitation to begin the spiritual journey that never ends. The author gives many examples drawn from his experience of the transforming power of this total approach to the human being.

This book can serve as a model for others who wish to integrate the medical, psychological, and spiritual-sacramental approaches to healing the whole person. This integration is desperately needed in Christian circles where these different aspects of our humanity have so often been separated. The author tells us that it can be done and is being done. Best of all, Dr. Bakken embodies the spiritual concern and caring of which this book speaks. Providing this kind of integration demands sacrifice and growth on the part of all those involved in bringing wholeness from potential to actuality, but the rewards are infinite.

MORTON KELSEY

Gualala, California

Acknowledgments

I would like to acknowledge and thank those important persons in my life who have been the inspiration for this book and who helped see it through to completion:

Theresa Appelö, my faithful and enduring wife, who has loved and nurtured me through my most difficult and painful times;

Robert Blair Ruble, pastor and friend, who believes in me and the vision I hold, and helped to establish St. Luke Health Ministries in reality;

Morton Kelsey, mentor and spiritual friend, who encouraged me to make the writing a priority;

Fran Cavey, friend and colleague, who carefully read and edited the manuscript and whose spirituality continually challenges me to set out into the deep;

St. Luke staff, board, and community, who have supported me with their unconditional love;

John Tivenan and Mary Kaye Willian, whose fresh insights in critiquing the manuscript helped mold the final format;

Martha List, who expertly edited and typed the words of the manuscript, but more importantly affirms the writer and the content;

Michael Leach and Frank Oveis, my editors, whose enthusiasm and suggestions helped make the process less painful.

I also wish to thank all those persons whose stories I have shared in love and gratitude but whose identities have been changed in the book to protect their privacy.

Introduction

This book has been written from a deep conviction that most Christians today have lost their way in life. For so many people, the church has failed "to bring good tidings to the afflicted" (Is 61:1). The words and tenets of our faith have become empty, pious rhetoric as we gather together on Sunday mornings—so often with a social-club mentality—expecting and receiving little. Well-being, transformation, freedom, wholeness—these seem as elusive as the Christ whom we profess as Lord. We have forgotten or lost the meaning of *living* the good news. We would do well to heed the scriptural call to wholeness: "I call heaven and earth to witness against you this day, that I have set before you life and death, blessing and curse; therefore, choose life, that you and your descendants may live" (Dt 30:19).

In our modern society we have turned to the helping professions, especially medicine, for most of the answers to the complex, life-denying problems (whether physical, psychological, or spiritual) that are confronted daily and which threaten to destroy. Very early in my professional career as a physician it became clear to me that thinly disguised behind the obvious problem (no matter what it is or how it presents itself) is a hurting *person* in search of healing, not just a cure. One does not need to probe very deeply to uncover the pain, the unforgiveness, the anger, the fear. But once revealed, what then is to be done? Traditionally, it has been far easier to prescribe a pill or some type of medical intervention rather than to deal with the root problems and the inevitable questions they engender. What does it mean to be healthy? Who or what controls my life? What brings me well-being and gives my life meaning?

1

What is the nature of reality and what is my role in it? What does it mean to be a whole person in the context of the gospel? Am I willing to change and grow? Do I choose life or death?

This book is meant both to nurture and to challenge those who believe, or would like to believe, that wholeness flows from a deep, Christ-centered spiritual commitment. The quality of a person's life journey is ultimately a reflection of his or her world view and spiritual odyssey. Of that I am certain. Therefore, these pages are more a pastoral letter of personal reflections on health and healing than a scholarly treatise. I have attempted to synthesize and integrate the glimpses of reality revealed in the physical, social, and health sciences with the truth of scripture revealed in the living Lord and experienced in lives transformed. I have tried to express in fresh ways the traditional message of the church, which for many people has become otherwise stale and void of any real meaning. From this unique perspective, my hope is that the many scriptural references cited will take on new significance and power.

There is a hunger for true health and a yearning for the life-giving, healing power of the gospel. The people of God can and must recapture, by the grace of God, whole and holy living *now*, not just in some nebulous future time.

Peace, joy, health!

KENNETH L. BAKKEN

Baltimore, Maryland

PART I

THE CHALLENGE: FEAR AS DESTROYER

But then what return did you get from the things
of which you are now ashamed?
The end of those things is death.

Romans 6:21

Chapter 1

Living in Neutral

I consider that the sufferings of this present time are not worth comparing with the glory that is to be revealed to us. For the creation waits with eager longing for the revealing of the sons of God.

Romans 8:18–19

Karen's family was told emphatically by the psychiatrists that she would probably never be well and might be functional only after eight to ten years of intensive psychotherapy and medication. I could not believe that my brilliant, beautiful friend was confined to a private psychiatric hospital, diagnosed as a paranoid schizophrenic, both homicidal and suicidal. I was confused, angry, and embarrassed. I denied the reality and the gravity of the situation; surely Karen would "snap out of it." After all, I thought, there was no history of mental illness in her family.

As a student beginning medical studies in the early 1970's, I researched books and sought out teachers and physicians in the vain hope that something had been overlooked, that there might be a medical breakthrough that would cure Karen of her affliction. Still she deteriorated, unable to fit into any reasonable pattern of normal family life. The family lived in constant fear and dread of Karen's violent outbursts and totally unpredictable, erratic, and often harmful behavior.

Karen's father was the pastor of a large church in California. Hundreds of people in the congregation and community and all over the country were praying for Karen's recovery, but it was as if God were absent from the scene. Where was this loving Lord whom we worshiped and served? Was there no compassion, no mercy?

Over two and one-half years of almost constant distress became nearly intolerable. This continuous crisis state was so much of a living hell that at times death became a more preferable option than life, not only for Karen but for all who were daily living her pain.

At this most bleak time, Karen's mother was reminded of a little book called *The Healing Light* written by an Episcopalian laywoman, Agnes Sanford. Karen's dad had read it years before during his seminary training and had dismissed it as "poor theology." It is a book about prayer and healing, written by a woman who believed that it is God's will that we be whole in body, mind, and spirit. Through prayer we can become channels of God's power and grace—the energy, the light that heals.

Out of desperation as much as God's leading, Karen's father wrote a letter to this woman who prayed for people. Serendipitously, Agnes lived in southern California within driving distance of their home. She invited Karen and the family to visit her, which they did. And from that initial time of loving presence and prayer with Mrs. Sanford, the Lord dramatically touched Karen and healed her of her disease. Agnes saw the fear and darkness that held her bound, commanded it to leave, and then prayed for the love and light and peace of God to fill her.

Karen's family, the psychiatrists, friends—all were astounded. The assumptions of our faith were challenged at their core; we could either change our world view or ignore the evidence. We chose to risk the danger of exploring this "burning bush." Had he not been inquisitive, Moses could have chosen to turn away from that bush not consumed by fire, and the Lord might well have left him to tend sheep the rest of his days. Karen's story, beautiful and powerful in its impact, is my burning bush.

The healing of my good friend Karen is an event that is singular in its profound influence on my life journey. Thus began, and still continues, an odyssey of conversion and transformation, a listening to that call to wholeness. Through the faith of one woman, Karen was called forth from premature death to life; I was being called from neutral living to growth, from the destructiveness of fear into the healing power of love.

Most people, however, live their entire lives in monotone. There is sound, but no rhythm or beat; there is color, but no vibrancy or pattern. God, self, and others remain hidden. We look, but do not see; we hear, but do not listen; we feel, but do not experience; we think, but do not understand. The burning bushes are never even approached. Dr. Frederick Franck, physician and author, offers his perspective as an artist in his book *The Zen of Seeing.*

> Millions of people, unseeing, joyless, bluster through life in their halfsleep, hitting, kicking and killing what they barely have perceived. They have never learned to see, or they have forgotten that man has eyes to see, to experience. When a man no longer experiences, the organs of his inner life wither away. Alone or in herds he goes on binges of violence and destruction.[1]

Jung observed that the human psyche seeks integration, that there is an instinctual drive toward wholeness and health. Very much as nature abhors a vacuum, the soul abhors separation and division. Yet in a fog of unawareness we often live in neutral, neither denying and disowning nor acknowledging and claiming. We wait for answers to be given rather than asking the questions that will make a difference. But St. Paul asks the ultimate question, making it clear who and what we are: "the sons [and daughters] of God" waiting eagerly for the glory that is being revealed to us (Rom 8:18–19). The burning bushes are all around us. The call is issued to holiness and wholeness, but we deny it, choosing rather our own path that leads ultimately to destruction.

A person must become aware of all the facets that contribute to healthy, "holy" living. Health is often viewed as merely the absence of disease or infirmity. Phrases such as "If I am not sick, then I must be healthy" imply neither a positive nor a negative state, simply a neutral one. The World Health Organization (WHO) more completely states that health is a "state of complete physical, mental, and social well-being." This operating definition is useful but has its drawbacks as well. It separates the person into physical, mental, and social components and completely omits the spiritual dimension. Recently, the Christian Medical Commission has encouraged and supported a world-wide examination by the churches of their own understanding of health. There has been widespread participation and exchange of ideas in regional conferences on this subject.

> Growing out of this study and reflection process has come a new formulation which suggests that health and wholeness as "a dynamic state of well-being of the individual and the society; of physical, mental, spiritual, economic, political and social well-being; of being in harmony with each other, with the natural environment and with God." Understood in this more dynamic sense of completeness, wholeness and harmony, health becomes a more meaningful goal.[2]

Health, then, is a term that is really very inclusive, but which is often used in a narrow sense and is confused with "medicine" and "medical care." Medicine is a part of health—both as a profession and a generic term. Medicine is practiced or administered both to alleviate sickness and suffering and to help cure a disease process in the restoration of health. Health, on the other hand, encompasses everything that has an impact on the human organism.

The relationship between medicine and health is often difficult to assess because most health indicators and statistics are not comprehensive but use only the "absence of disease" definition. If we consider the health of entire populations and the health of society in general, medical interventions have had little impact or effect. By and large the improved life expectancy at birth for Americans over the past one hundred years can be credited primarily to activities that include environmental improvements, safe housing and water supplies, waste disposal, regulations in food safety, and immunization programs. These programs have had their primary effects on the reduction of infant and childhood mortality. Just one of these simple prevention and promotion measures probably has more influence on our health than all the hospital beds in the United States. But the public, as well as the medical establishment, tends to idolize high technology—high-cost hospital care—in the name of health. The biomedical model, with its primary focus on disease care and crisis intervention, is necessary and good. But it must be placed within the wider context and perspective of health.

Today, public health statistics show that how long we live is not the problem but rather the quality of life. Over the past fifty years there has been a changing pattern of disease entities with a dramatic decline in the age-adjusted mortality rates. There is also a concomitant increase in chronic illness. Persons with chronic problems now constitute more than sixty percent of all admissions to hospitals and more than fifty percent of all physician visits. This dramatic increase in long-term, chronic, disabling, severe illness along with a tremendous increase in the elderly population, especially over 85 years of age, constitute major factors challenging our social fabric.[3]

Average per diem hospital rates, which include just room, board, and nursing care, have increased at twice the rate of inflation. Hospitals take more than forty percent of the available health care dollars. Medical care has become big business: health insurance practices discourage individual responsibility, and the number of practicing physicians has doubled. This big-business mentality combined with societal changes such as increased mobility, increase in single-parent homes, and greater sexual freedom underscores a key missing element— human love and support. Caring and compassion must begin to take precedence over competition if we truly seek *health* for our people and the people of the world.[4]

In a practical and delightful book, *The Wellness Workbook*, John Travis describes our state of health as the tip of an iceberg rising above the surface of the water. There are other levels below this tip, such as life-style behaviors and psychological makeup, that influence our state of health. Deeper yet in the broadening base of the iceberg are the spiritual, philosophical, and transpersonal realms, to which we can add the world view and paradigms out of which we consciously, subconsciously (or preconsciously), and unconsciously operate. Dr. Travis elucidates that at this deepest level the concerns become

> such issues as reason for being, our place in the universe. It is the attending to or not attending to such questions, that underlies and permeates all of the layers above, and ultimately determines whether the tip of the iceberg, representing our state of health, is one of disease or wellness.[5]

When we lack sufficient awareness of these aspects of life that contribute to our total well-being, health eludes us. We live in neutral. Creativity is often squelched, and responses become rote. As in the case of my friend Karen we find ourselves physically, mentally, and spiritually in a downward spiral toward disease, disintegration, and premature death.

Jerry, a 38-year-old businessman, presented himself one afternoon at the St. Luke Health Center. That morning he had begun to experience a "racing" heart, pressure in his chest, excessive sweating, and weakness in his legs. My immediate response as a physician was to determine whether he was, in fact, experiencing a myocardial infarction—a heart attack. An electrocardiogram was run and found to be normal; blood was drawn and sent to the laboratory for immediate evaluation. Physical examination revealed a man who was thirty pounds overweight with a slightly elevated blood pressure and pulse rate. But it was in talking with Jerry that real insights into his problem began to emerge.

He had been to emergency rooms and medical clinics previously with similar signs and symptoms. He even recognized his general anxiety. But no one had ever helped him connect his internal, vague feelings of depression, despair, and impending doom with the external physical manifestations. Jerry lived most of life in neutral, very much unaware of the whole of the iceberg that permeated his state of health. After gentle probing, he revealed the underlying problems. He ate too much of the wrong kinds of food and drank too much alcohol. He had stopped his regular running program. His business was deteriorating, and his finances were so precarious that he would soon need to sell his house. His marriage had deteriorated to the point of talk of separation and divorce. Religion did not play an active role in his existence.

Jerry had been seeking a "quick fix"—a "please-take-it-all-from-me" magical potion. He was living life failing to see, comprehend, experience, and learn with the inevitable destructive outcomes that brings. He was living in neutral.Through a willingness to be vulnerable and to change, he began to seek health. Jerry found himself and a God who loves him and wishes to dwell with and in him.

According to the American Academy of Family Physicians, two-thirds of office visits to family doctors are prompted by stress-related symptoms (like Jerry's). Basically, when we are subjected to major stress (or distress), we are aroused to a "fight or flight" reaction[6], because information received from the perception of either internal or external stimuli cause both neurophysiological and emotional/psychological responses. Unlike animals, we most often cannot fight or flee, although our inclination may be to do one or the other. Kenneth Pelletier, in his book *Mind as Healer, Mind as Slayer*, describes a common reaction:

> In our complex society with its highly refined codes of acceptable behavior, fighting and fleeing are often not considered appropriate reactions to stressful situations. When your boss informs you that you will not receive the raise in salary you expected, you cannot physically assault him, nor can you literally run away from the situation. Therefore, you muster all your resources to respond in a dignified manner and internalize your distress. However, your body is en-

tering into a state of stress preparedness, despite your en-
forced outward calm. Messages are transmitted throughout
the neuroendocrine system which cause significant changes
in your biochemistry . . . Our neurophysical responses for
dealing with stress have become anachronistic. Since society dictates that the standard modes of stress-release behavior are unacceptable, and since the nature of our social
organization places such an unprecedented amount of stress
upon each individual in the society, many of us sustain pro-
longed stress responses far more frequently than is condu-
cive to health maintenance.[7]

Stress is known to be a major contributor, either directly or
indirectly, to coronary heart disease, cancer, lung ailments, ac-
cidental injuries, cirrhosis of the liver and suicide—six of the
leading causes of death in the United States. Stress also plays a
role in aggravating such disease conditions as diabetes, arthri-
tis, multiple sclerosis, and genital herpes. Our life-style seems
to be a principal cause of many illnesses. The three most pre-
scribed drugs in this country—Tagamet for peptic ulcers, In-
deral for high blood pressure, and Valium for anxiety—offer a
sad commentary on the way we have chosen to live as individuals and as a society. We are living in neutral.

The relentless stresses of poverty and ghetto life are also associated with higher health risks. Studies of poor black neigh-
borhoods in Detroit and Boston have correlated high blood
pressure with overcrowded housing and high levels of unemployment and crime. The prevalence of hypertension among
American blacks is generally twice that of whites.

A single event like losing a job can have a ripple effect, caus-
ing other changes that touch every aspect of existence. The
greatest source of stress may not be the actual loss of the job
but rather the gradual domestic and psychological changes it
imposes. These can be devastating according to Harvey Brenner, a sociologist at the Johns Hopkins University School of
Hygiene and Public Health. Dr. Brenner has found that over a
period of about twenty-five years beginning in the late 1940's,
for each 1 percent increase in the national unemployment rate,

there were 1.9 percent more U.S. deaths from heart disease and cirrhosis, 4.1 percent more suicides, and an upturn in the number of first-time admissions to state mental-health facilities (up 4.3 percent for men, 2.3 percent for women).[8]

Individually and collectively we make choices that keep us living in neutral. The nuclear arms race with the real possibility of annihilation of the human family is a major documented psychological stress factor in every person's life. The insanity of the arms race is underscored by the fact that even the most avid hawks do not believe in the eventualities against which we are spending billions of dollars. We are blinded by hate and obsessed with a Soviet threat when we should be collectively creating new approaches to the massive problems that confront us as a people—industrial collapse, energy crises, inadequate or nonexistent health care, political paralysis, and world-wide starvation.

A major problem of nuclear power is the disposal of nuclear waste. Tons of waste are produced annually by the building of nuclear weapons and by the fuel of each nuclear reactor. The most poisonous is plutonium; it is the most dangerous, the most long-lived, and remains toxic for five-hundred thousand years. This is the length of time that plutonium must be isolated from the environment. A release of only a small amount of plutonium (less than one pound) world-wide could theoretically cause cancer in every man, woman, and child. Storage and disposal of nuclear waste is a volatile concern if for no other reason than that some of our major industries have not even been trustworthy about properly containing, sealing, and storing toxic chemicals, which are far less dangerous than nuclear waste. I need only cite Love Canal in New York State and hundreds of other dump sites around the country and the deleterious health effects they have had. Do we have the moral right to contaminate the earth with deadly nuclear waste for thousands of generations to come? It is often a question of greed, power, and control. Many scientists contend that solar technology is sufficiently advanced to be economically and practically feasible. Yet nuclear technology is heavily promoted because it is an energy source that leads to a high concentration of economic and political power for a small elite. These are unprecedented threats posed by nuclear technology and the arms race. It should be "abundantly clear to anyone that it is unsafe, uneconomical, irresponsible, and immoral: totally unacceptable."[9] It is living in neutral.

We are challenged to identify with the poor by a concrete relationship. But even while living and working in West Africa and Central America, I had a tendency to isolate myself from the shock of the overwhelming problems confronted on a daily basis. It was much easier to dine with a member of the diplomatic corps or spend the day at a hotel swimming pool than to stand in solidarity with the impoverished and oppressed people I had come to serve. But proximity can breed compassion and understanding as we begin gradually to hear the cry of the poor in their vulnerability and wretched condition. With enlightened eyes we read the words of St. John, "But if anyone has the world's goods and sees his brother in need, yet closes his heart against him, how does God's love abide in him?" (I Jn 3:17).

It is important to begin to comprehend the needs of our brothers and sisters in manageable terms of comparison. If the world were a village of 100 people, 70 of them would be unable to read, over 50 would be suffering from malnutrition, and over 80 would live in what we call substandard housing. Of the 100 members of the global village, 6 would be Americans. These 6 would have one-half of the village's entire income and would consume one-third of the total energy resources available. Of the 6 Americans, less than 2 percent would own 80 percent of the U.S. corporate wealth. That is living in neutral.

My experiences as an international health-care worker in Ghana and Guatemala are mirrored in most large cities in the U.S. as well as in rural America. Literally surrounding many of the finest medical institutions in this country one encounters devastating poverty. Crime, unemployment, and infant mortality rates are all appallingly high. It is unbelievable that schools of medicine and public health often have had little or no impact on the incredible health and social problems present at their collective doorsteps. The priorities involved are obvious: competition rather than compassion and an obsession with sophisticated technology over pressing human need. That is living in neutral.

In the rotunda of the Johns Hopkins Hospital stands an immense marble statue of Jesus—*Christus Consolator,* the Divine Healer—with arms outstretched in beckoning love. The inscription on the base reads, "Come unto me, all ye that are weary and are heavy laden, and I will give you rest" (Mt 11:28, KJV). This verse continues in the Gospel of St. Matthew, "Take my yoke upon you, and learn from me; for I am gentle and lowly in heart, and you will find rest for your souls." This Jesus who calls us to himself also impels us to learn from him—this Lord who is gentle and humble. If those of us who teach and work in these places dedicated to the care of the sick would more fully yoke ourselves to the Christ, how much lighter the load would be! We would become a loving, nurturing, human community promoting health: justice, wholeness, and peace.

Jim Wallis, founder of the Sojourners community in Washington, D.C., challenges us to understand the implications of living in neutral as a society:

> The anxiety-ridden and the poverty-stricken are two major segments of humanity in the world today. To recognize this fact is to acknowledge the truth of the oppressor-oppressed division but to go beyond class consciousness to spiritual consciousness . . .
>
> The result of prosperity based on injustice is anxiety. Gloom, cynicism, despair, and hedonism are all fruits of the fundamental anxiety that characterizes the cultures of the wealthy nations. The spiritual crisis of the rich countries directly corresponds to the economic crisis of the poor countries. The rich hunger in spirit while the poor hunger for bread. Our spiritual malaise is the consequence of affluence in the face of deprivation. Conversion in our time is to liberate the poor and to make the blind see. The poor need justice, and the rich need restored sight.[10]

Living in a society that rewards material success, our worth is often measured as a function of our accomplishments and acquisitions rather than *who* we are as persons. The church has also been guilty of perpetuating this fallacious thinking and neutral living. If we worship in a beautiful sanctuary, have a large, active membership, and promote many different programs during the week, then we are considered successful and blessed. I have often asked myself the question: *If* I secure the proper academic degrees, teach at a prestigious university, engage in full-time health ministry, and provide well for my family, *then* am I successful? I might even exclaim with the Prophet Elijah, "I have been very jealous for the Lord, the God of hosts . . ." (1 Kgs 19:10). But Elijah's success in defeating and then destroying the priests of Baal was very short-lived indeed. Queen Jezebel sought to kill him; he was afraid and fled for his life.

Often we are afraid and want to flee, to escape the overwhelming anxiety and pressures of life. We, too, have sat down under a "broom tree" and have wanted to give up. How fleeting is the joy in the "successes." Elijah became discouraged and depressed; he wanted to die. He didn't want to eat or drink, and he hid in a mountain cave. But the word of the Lord came to him in his weakness and vulnerability.

> And he said, "Go forth, and stand upon the mount before the Lord." And, behold, the Lord passed by, and a great and strong wind rent the mountains, and broke in pieces the rocks before the Lord, but the Lord was not in the wind; and after the wind an earthquake, but the Lord was not in the earthquake; and after the earthquake a fire, but the Lord was not in the fire; and after the fire a still small voice. (1 Kgs 19:11–12)

Elijah was probably prepared for something spectacular, like the show of awesome power on Mount Carmel when the altars and priests of Baal were consumed by fire. But the Lord came to him in a whisper. Often in our lowest moments of neutral living, perhaps in the still solitude of the late night, God seeks to touch us, as he touched Karen. God sought him in the quiet prayer of a faithful woman.

Lord, we are ready to listen; heighten our awareness to the cries of your people. "Bring forth the people who are blind, yet have eyes, who are deaf, yet have ears!" (Is 43:8).

Chapter 2

Disease, Disintegration, and Death

> Do you not know that you are God's temple and that
> God's Spirit dwells in you?
>
> *1 Corinthians 3:16*

W hen I was an intern at a teaching hospital in Seattle, Washington, I was surrounded by disease. I lived in its midst most of my waking hours. Trained as a technician in curative care, the thought of stemming this onslaught of sickness of body, mind—and, most assuredly, spirit—sometimes seemed overwhelming. In fact, it became that. I often hated this my chosen profession. And I sometimes feared it as much for the power it wielded as for the responsibility it engendered.

When a person would come to the outpatient clinic or emergency room complaining of a chronically elevated fever, productive cough, blood-tinged sputum, and chest pain, my job was to provide a medical intervention to alleviate the suffering and treat the immediate problem—possibly pneumonia by the signs and symptoms described. During the two or three weeks prior to the medical examination, the runny nose, sneezing, general malaise, achiness, and cough may have been recognized by the afflicted person as a simple cold and treated as such at home. But when the condition changed and worsened, help was sought. Likewise, simple stomach upset that persisted and developed into sharp abdominal pains, black, tarry stools, and persistent vomiting would cause a person to seek the advice of a health practitioner. Similarly, mental depression that became a chronic condition in which the person began to consider taking his/her own life would be a crisis situation needing intervention. In each of the above examples, the familiar becomes the unknown, and the fear of our own mortality grips us with the prospects of disease and death. The implications of a cold versus pneumonia are very different. A person can hemorrhage and die from peptic ulcer disease. Feeling "down" for a few days is obviously much less serious than becoming suicidally depressed for weeks or months.

Signs and symptoms are those things that can be observed by the individual or by someone else; they should be viewed as important clues. They demand attention; they provide warning signals and often act as a gauge of our health or lack of health. Signs and symptoms that persist may be indicative of a disease process (physical, mental, or spiritual) that may, in fact, be life-threatening. *Dis-ease* is the absence of ease. It is a breakdown in communication of the systems in the body, in which the physical, mental, and spiritual needs of the person are not being expressed in a way that is unique to self. There is failure in adapting to life.

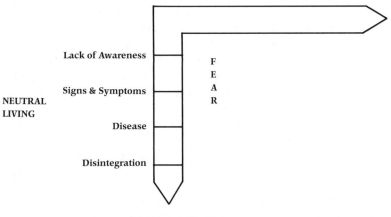

PREMATURE DEATH

In the vertical "neutral living" axis of this model,[1] the human organism begins to deteriorate toward a premature death when the disease does not respond to the full biomedical armamentarium offered. Disintegration of bodily and mental functions leads ultimately to death for everyone. The early church thought of death as synonymous with evil and saw it inflicting damage in three major ways: (1) morally on other people, (2) mentally on ourselves, and (3) physically on ourselves. The resurrection of the Christ, on the other hand, is viewed as the defeat of Death. We are set free from its bondage both in this life and in the hereafter.

But in the modern medical setting, the ultimate existential question of death is rarely addressed and is, in fact, avoided as much as possible as a result of a Cartesian world view,[2] which is discussed in chapters three and four. Physicist and author Fritjof Capra writes:

> The lack of spirituality that has become characteristic of our modern technological society is reflected in the fact that the medical profession, like society as a whole, is death-denying. Within the mechanistic framework of our medical science, death cannot be qualified. The distinction between a good death and a poor death does not make sense; death becomes simply the total standstill of the body machine.[3]

However, we read in the scriptures that the Word became flesh—body. This living Word, Jesus—the divine presence in and through human flesh—was tortured and put to death. But in the resurrection his body was restored and stands uniquely as a glorious witness to the wholeness of our being. Resurrection, then, and its promise of life, also relates inextricably to the question of death.

Death *can* be qualified. During his ministry, Jesus resurrected three persons from death—Jairus's daughter (Mk 5), the widow's son (Lk 7), and his friend Lazarus (Jn 11). These stories deal with *premature* death; these were young people. But after each was restored to life, he/she died again in the fullness of time. Premature death as opposed to death with full years or death in the fullness of time are quite different in the Bible. Moses died (with full sexual potency) by the kiss of the mouth of God at a full, old age. Lazarus, the widow's son, and Jairus's daughter did not. Their deaths were premature and were, therefore, an affront to God's purposes. Jesus confronted this distortion of life and responded in his healing ministry.

Jesus' task is to reconcile all that is separated and alienated from the Father. "And I, when I am lifted up from the earth, will draw all men to myself" (Jn 12:32). It is beyond our own power to do so. But Jesus resurrects, restores, and renews, and we can celebrate the ongoing incarnation of God in all that is love through our brothers and sisters.

The root cause of our alienation is fear. Fear is the motivating or propelling force that keeps us fragmented and living in neutral. We are closed to the love of God revealed decisively in the Christ and brought continuously to us embodied in human presence. James Nelson, in his controversial book, *Embodiment*, states that theology in the Christian West "has too often been a disembodied enterprise."[4] He writes about the "body-self," a term pointing to the unity of the person and the significance of incarnation, communion, desire, and feeling. We must *feel* in our whole bodies—rationally, emotionally, and spiritually—if we are really to perceive and know anything.

> The term body-self. . . . is the refusal to be split into mind over body over heart over head. It is the refusal to locate true selfhood in only part of the self. The notion of feeling, then, is one way of pointing to the unified response of the body-self. And unified response means listening to the messages from all dimensions of the self—the mind, the heart, the spiritual senses, the genitals, the viscera.[5]

Desire is also an expression of the body-self. We open ourselves to God desiring to receive. "Not to desire is not to receive, and not to receive is not to know. But, conversely, to desire can mean to know, and to know can mean to love."[6] In true communion with God and with one another we can experience participation and unity rather than possession and competition.

Out of fear we deny our bodies as really meaningful or worthwhile—it is my heart or my blood vessels that are sick, not my whole person, of which my heart and vessels are an integral part. The body carries all the meaningful content of our lives. Depth psychologist Ira Progoff notes that our body is the physical counterpart of our whole life history. It is our way of experiencing the life process most meaningfully. Our lack of total self-acceptance, including full awareness of our sexuality and of knowing God's unconditional acceptance of us, keeps us from truly embracing genuine wholeness. We deny the "wisdom of the body." To accept the heretical trichotomy of body/mind/spirit is to allow "fate" (in Christian terms, evil) to run its course until crisis intervention no longer is tenable and death claims us prematurely. As followers of Jesus, we can break this destructive downward spiral. We are invited by Nelson into the full meaning of the first chapter of St. John's Gospel.

> But the Word did become flesh. Logos, Cosmic Meaning, was embodied, and our own embodiment has been given definition and vindication in Jesus Christ. What is at stake . . . is whether or not it is possible, however partially we may expe-.rience it, that there be a genuine and deeply personal union of God and our embodied selves. If we deny the radicality of God's incarnation in Jesus, we may well persist in a vain attempt to be more spiritual than God. The possibility of our own full humanity, after all, decisively hinges upon "the humanity of God" (to use Karl Barth's fine phrase) . . . In those central symbols of incarnation and resurrection Christian faith affirms that God embraces fleshly, bodily life. God invites us to do so.[7]

When we do *not* do so, we embrace a spirituality that fosters flight from the world and suppresses the body as the enemy. We become disembodied spirits, and loneliness, depressive guilt feelings, alienation, and anger lead us farther away from the growth and freedom of the completeness we so desperately seek. This became poignantly clear to me during my internship year. One man's struggle in particular remains etched in my memory.

On an early fall morning as I reviewed patient charts, I was told by one of the nurses that a new patient had arrived on the floor the previous evening. When I entered this man's room I was struck by the softball-size swelling in his neck, which I soon learned had been diagnosed as thyroid cancer. He related to me that his cancer had been preceded by a history of chronic psychological stress and several severe life-change events, including a recent divorce. Significant precursors of the discovery of the tumor included anxiety, depression, hopelessness, and grief. Throughout his entire life he had felt impotent to change. Now his worst fears were being played out; he said he was dying of cancer.

As I completed the customary duties of an intern—a thorough medical history and physical examination—I became aware of a "still small voice" within me that was urging me to pray for this man with the enlarged, cancerous thyroid. Pray? Do a history and physical examination, talk with him, counsel him about his illness perhaps, order tests and specialists—yes. But pray? The deep intuitive movement within me persisted, and I began to bargain with God. I said, "Lord, I know all about prayer and healing intellectually, and certainly by my intimate experience with my friend Karen. But, Lord, you don't understand. This is a hospital and this man has cancer. I don't have enough faith for this kind of thing. What good would I do?" And so the dialogue continued that morning as I completed my rounds.

I was reticent, as an intern especially, to talk with *any* patients about God, let alone pray with them. Would I be presumptuous to think that Jesus might want me to minister to the sick in prayer as well as through medication and surgery? What if the attending physicians discovered my covert "therapy"? What would I do if I were dismissed from the intern training program? These fears and other questions leaped through my mind and subconsciously begged to be challenged. I knew that the Lord was the healer and that I could only facilitate the process of restoration of health. By afternoon I had forgotten about it.

That evening my wife questioned me about my distracted restlessness. I brushed her comments aside as intern's syndrome—chronic anxiety and exhaustion. In bed at an early hour, I again heard the still small voice within, and God's presence seemed very near. I did not sleep well as I wrestled with its meaning. Actually, I wanted to escape; I wanted to push it all away from me. By morning I had again forgotten about my encounter; my list of details for the day filled my conscious mind.

I arrived at the hospital earlier than usual. It was quiet when I walked onto the ward, and I was immediately struck with the feeling that I had some unfinished business with God. "All right, Lord, you win. But no one will ever know that I did this." The man with the thyroid tumor was sitting up in bed, as if he had been expecting me at 6:30 A.M. After greeting him I asked if I might palpate his neck because, I explained, I would be presenting his case during rounds that afternoon. I had decided beforehand that this was an appropriate cover for a quick, surreptitious, silent prayer. As I stood behind the man and placed my fingers over his enlarged thyroid, I tried to remember what I had learned from Agnes Sanford and my uncle.[8] I praised God for being present; I asked him to use me as his instrument; I visualized the healing power of God flowing into the tumor and shrinking it; I imagined the man well, as God had intended; I thanked the Lord that he had heard me and that I could depend on his promises.

I stood there for what seemed like a long time. I worried that the patient might think I was strange. I wanted to appear competent and in control, and I certainly did not want him to know I was praying for him. I departed, relieved that it was over and that the Lord could now leave me alone. There were more important, life-saving things to be done in the hospital that day.

In my usual busyness, the afternoon came quickly. It was time for rounds with the attending physician, resident, medical student, nurse, another intern, and myself. In the hallway outside the room of the man with the thyroid cancer, I vaguely wondered if any changes had occurred since the morning. I presented his case in the typical medical tradition, and the entourage entered the room. I will never forget the expression of surprise on the internist's face as he asked, "*What* happened to you?" The man answered nonchalantly that he had noticed that the tumor had been gradually shrinking as the day had progressed. The thyroid had shrunk from the size of a softball to the size of a Ping-Pong ball in about six hours! I was awed and delighted, but I did not say a word.

The next day the patient was transferred to an oncology center for further tests and treatment. My hectic schedule precluded any follow-up. And it was just as well that it happened that way. I had prayed more out of obedience and hope than out of a faith that was certain that something would happen. But deep inside me I know he was healed of his disease. Since then I have never questioned the Lord's promptings in prayer again. I spend greater time listening now, with one ear directed toward God and the other to the person in need. I have moved several steps further out of neutral living.

This man with the cancer experienced the signs and symptoms of his disease. He had deteriorated to a critical point and was approaching death at age fifty. He was afraid, but I could be for him the Lord's embrace of unconditional acceptance, which says, "My love is for everyone; it is also for you." My hope is that he began to get in touch with the many repressed inner dimensions that were left unexplored. In his ministry, Jesus called forth these areas in many people.

Jesus never ignored a person's deepest needs, feelings, and desires. The gospel accounts record many examples. At the pool of Bethsaida Jesus asked the man who had been sick for thirty-eight years if he wanted to be healed (Jn 5). For many people it is preferable and easier to remain sick within the disease model we have presented than it is to change. In the story of the paralytic lowered through the roof by faithful friends, Jesus chooses to forgive the man's sins first, so that the physical healing might be significant and complete (Mk 2). We see Jesus calling forth from the crowd the woman with the hemorrhage who told him the whole truth of her life, probably revealing the most intimate details of her signs, symptoms, disease, and subsequent disintegration. Only after this does Jesus dismiss her in wholeness (Mk 5). The Samaritan woman at the well was called to acknowledgment (Jn 4). Jesus asked the blind beggar Bartimaeus, "What do you want me to do for you?" (Mk 10:51). We, too, are asked if we really want to get well, to acknowledge the painful truth of our lives, and what we might desire of the Lord. We must begin to answer these difficult questions in order to move out of the neutral living—premature death axis.

Jesus also confronted the societal structures that trap so many people in a downward, disease-oriented spiral. Individual and collective disease and disintegration are often the result of duplicity and are the opposite of a natural, unselfconscious openness, which is simplicity. Richard Foster calls simplicity an inward reality that results in an outward life-style.[9] He challenges us to begin to free ourselves from the tyranny of things, of self and others. Simplicity is often the fruit of other disciplines such as solitude and silence, prayer and meditation, forgiveness and confession, guidance and submission. When our lives are not open in these ways to the grace and mercy of God, we are neither simple nor free. In fact, we often become sick in spirit, mind, and body.

The signs and symptoms of such societal diseases as racism, militarism, sexism, and nationalism are obvious and prevalent. Our collective disintegration and premature death may come in the form of the majority of our resources being diverted to preparation for war and then finally ultimate destruction by nuclear holocaust. Analogously, as individuals we clamor for self-recognition and attention. We create an environment of pretentiousness and material possessions. We bind ourselves in greed and hostility. Our life-style is killing us, literally and figuratively.

Instead of a sickness-producing dependence upon our own devices, we are called to a radical dependence upon God for everything. "Behold, to the Lord your God belong heaven and the heaven of heavens, the earth with all that is in it" (Dt 10:14). We are accountable for God's generosity to us. We are commanded to give freely, as we have received freely, trusting that God will always provide for our needs. There can be no true wholeness, well-being, peace *(shalom)* without justice, the call *to* wholeness *(mishpat)*. We are a people who cling to our weapons rather than to our God for security; we insulate and isolate ourselves from the poor; we destroy the creation—earth, water, and air—with every manner of poison; and we serve the rival god of *mammon* above the God of love and compassion. Justice is demanded first before true individual and collective health and wholeness are possible. This challenges the core of our affluent life-style.

The Christ event, the Day of the Lord, establishes the age to come as already among us. The power of God has broken into human history. We should live scandalously free. We don't need to watch out for "number one" because we have one who watches out for us. The central point is to seek *first* the kingdom and then everything else will come in its proper order, including health.

Listen anew to the words of the Apostle Paul:

> Not that I complain of want; for I have learned, in whatever state I am, to be content. I know how to be abused, and I know how to abound; in any and all circumstances I have learned the secret of facing plenty and hunger, abundance and want. I can do all things in him who strengthens me. (Phil 4:11–13)

The disintegration of self and society is propelled by fear. Love and hope are limited where fear predominates. When love and hope are no longer a powerful influence, we wither and die. We cannot function normally and effectively without expectation and belief in fulfillment; we become severely impaired without hope. When hope is lost, the will to live also slips away and the phenomenon of rapidly ensuing death is well known to everyone. Even more striking is a phenomenon known in Australia, where an aboriginal person, on seeing what he or she interprets as a vision of his or her own death in the eyes of another, may yield completely to the inevitability of death and, in a very short time, simply die.

The absence of hope and confidence can contravene many positive efforts to bring about healing. This is true for individuals as well as for groups of people. In the case of cancer, it has been hypothesized that unresolved guilt and grief lead to a breakdown of the body's immune mechanisms, which is probably the key to rejecting many incipient malignant processes normally. The "cancers" of our society need an infusion of hope, through conversion, before they metastasize and cause death. In our faith as Christians "we rejoice in our *hope* of sharing the glory of God" (Rom 5:2).

Dr. Stuart Kingma, former director of the Christian Medical Commission of the World Council of Churches, writes of yet another dimension of human existence that is important in the support of hope:

> . . . This relates to the social and communal dimension of what it is to be human, the undergirding of those around us who love and touch our lives. To be human is to be "in community," to see ourselves as neighbours, interdependent, living together, accessible and perhaps even living for the other. People are tactile, sensuous, loving and social beings; we like to touch and to be touched. Hope and confidence and a positive current in our lives is maintained when we feel this solidarity with those around us and are comfortable with our role in that. This solidarity finds its expression in sharing, being a healing element within that community and supporting the identity of those around us (and in turn being supported in this way). The very ill, the dying, the elderly and infirm, and those with disfiguring or disabling conditions, draw strength from the warm and ready touch of those who visit them, the touch that speaks of acceptance, of giving, of caring.[10]

If we cannot draw upon the intimacy and strength of a loving community, especially a community of faith, there is an intense feeling of loneliness and isolation that affects health. Loneliness is a serious malady that cuts across every cultural, social, racial, and economic line.

> Loneliness and lack of companionship are the greatest unrecognized contributors to premature death in the United

States today . . . People who live alone—single, widowed, divorced—have death rates from two to ten times higher than those of individuals who live with others. Living alone is not the same as loneliness, but the two are often related.[11]

We all suffer; it is part of the human condition. We all die; that, too, is human. But St. Paul's words ring full and true:

> . . . We rejoice in our sufferings, knowing that suffering produces endurance, and endurance produces character, and character produces hope, and hope does not disappoint us, because God's love has been poured into our hearts through the Holy Spirit which has been given to us. (Rom 5:3–5)

PART II

THE INVITATION: LOVE AS MENDER

There is no fear in love,
but perfect love casts out fear.

1 John 4:18

Chapter 3
Living in Awareness

> . . . that they should seek God, in the hope that they might feel after him and find him. Yet he is not far from each one of us, for "In him we live and move and have our being"; as even some of your poets have said, "For we are indeed his offspring."
>
> *Acts 17:27–28*

We are faced with a crisis the proportions of which are just beginning to be realized by the medical, theological, and socio-political structures and institutions world wide. There is a crisis of confidence not only in the persons in leadership positions but also in the failing solutions to increasingly urgent needs. The daily litany of crime, disease, starvation, war, threat of nuclear destruction, inflation, and pollution, to name a few, is lethal to the human person. This lack of confidence certainly can deaden any creative responses, as we simply and unthinkingly mouth stock answers based upon a world view that is no longer valid.

Physicist Fritjof Capra is one prophetic voice; he sees the problems as systemic, which means that they are closely interconnected and interdependent.

> They cannot be understood within the fragmented methodology characteristic of our academic disciplines and government agencies. Such an approach will never resolve any of our difficulties but will merely shift them around in the complex web of social and ecological relations. A resolution can be found only if the structure of the web itself is changed, and this will involve profound transformations of our social institutions, values, and ideas.[1]

We give answers before we ask the questions—questions that can make a difference in how we live and how we perceive ourselves and our world. A question opens up the space wherein a difference can emerge. What can be said at the level of understanding, in giving answers, is not the whole reality. To take responsibility for oneself and to think for oneself is to live within an open question. We must begin to ask the questions that will lead to reconciliation and healing, individually and corporately, and ensure the survival of our planet.

The problems that we face cannot be solved by thinking more of the same. The paradigm, the space or question, must change. A space must be created where something more powerful can be revealed. To live life in the power of a question opens up possibilities that otherwise remain hidden. We need to bring forth the questions that can make a difference in our individual lives as well as in our institutions and organizations. The answers that have been provided, to do it better or differently, are variations on the same theme and have kept us trapped in a world that is rapidly changing and in a world view long since obsolete. What was once the product of visionaries is now the only thing that is practical. Personal and public egos must be put aside. Opinions and beliefs must be suspended in order to ask the necessary questions.

What is the ultimate question? The question that must be asked is: "What is wholeness and how is it attained?" When we really begin to ask what in life brings us meaning and fullness, peace, joy, and all the fruits of the Spirit, we joltingly discover that the current answers of "better" or "differently" miss the mark. As a people and society proud of its economic and technological achievements, we somehow think that more of the same can and will fix things up. We have equated our identity with our rational mind rather than with our whole being. This emphasis on rational thought in our culture is epitomized in Descartes's celebrated statement, *Cogito, ergo sum*—"I think, therefore I am."

Healing and well-being to most have become a visit to a practitioner or the hospital to be "treated," or newer and improved instruments of destruction in the name of defense in order to "feel safe," or more consumer commodities to be "comfort-able." But an honest look at the question reveals that healing is the call to wholeness. It is the dynamic equivalent of the cosmic dance: symbol, metaphor, myth. To assign healing a literal, one-dimensional meaning (such as disease-oriented curative care in a highly sophisticated setting) is to shrink and stifle and distort its significance. Rational thinking is linear, whereas an ecological awareness of healing and wholeness arises from an intuition of nonlinear systems such as movement and dance.

Healing, expressed in terms of the movement of the Creator in the universe, trembles with a sense of inexpressible mystery, a mystery that nevertheless addresses us in the totality of our being. The physicists and mathematicians themselves no longer speak of a literal, mechanistic, objectively quantifiable reality. Rather they stand in awe of the wonder and the interdependence and interconnectedness of all creation. Capra explains this within its historical context in his notable book *The Turning Point:*

> Since the seventeenth century physics has been the shining example of an "exact" science, and has served as the model for all other sciences. For two and a half centuries physicists have used a mechanistic view of the world to develop and refine the conceptual framework known as classical physics. They have based their ideas on the mathematical theory of Isaac Newton, the philosophy of René Descartes, and the scientific methodology advocated by Francis Bacon, and developed them in accordance with the general conception of reality prevalent during the seventeenth, eighteenth, and nineteenth centuries. Matter was thought to be the basis of all existence, and the material world was seen as a multitude of separate objects assembled into a huge machine. Like human-made machines, the cosmic machine was thought to consist of elementary parts. Consequently it was believed that complex phenomena could always be understood by reducing them to their basic building blocks and by looking for the mechanisms through which these interacted. This attitude, known as reductionism, has become so deeply ingrained in our culture that it has often been identified with

the scientific method. The other sciences accepted the mechanistic and reductionistic views of classical physics as the correct description of reality and modeled their own theories accordingly. Whenever psychologists, sociologists, or economists wanted to be scientific, they naturally turned toward the basic concepts of Newtonian physics.

In the twentieth century, however, physics has gone through several conceptual revolutions that clearly reveal the limitations of the mechanistic world view and lead to an organic, ecological view of the world which shows great similarities to the views of the mystics of all ages and traditions. The universe is no longer seen as a machine, made up of a multitude of separate objects, but appears as a harmonious indivisible whole; a network of dynamic relationships that include the human observer and his or her consciousness in an essential way. The fact that modern physics, the manifestation of an extreme specialization of the rational mind, is now making contact with mysticism, the essence of religion and manifestation of an extreme specialization of the intuitive mind, shows very beautifully the unity and complementary nature of the rational and intuitive modes of consciousness.[2]

The best minds in physics are saying that they do not know enough about matter to say that spirit is not, and that they can never provide a complete and definitive description of reality. The scientific theories will always be approximations to the true nature of things. The truth of reality can come only through spiritual revelation as it interpenetrates the physical in innumerable ways. "Spirituality speaks of the Spirit of God who reveals and manifests himself as source of life, freedom, and love within the totality which is the human person and his or her world and history."[3] Reality is not static or stagnant; it bristles with meanings and possibilities. But to live in this growing awareness we must open ourselves to a world view that is not maintained by dogmatism and misguided loyalties. What we have no world view to see, we do not even perceive. Healing will become an exaggeration, a fetish, or a sentimentality if there is no world view to support it. Spirituality becomes words rather than a life-style of gospel discipleship. We remain caught in a downward spiral of unawareness in neutral living.

The old paradigm comprises ideas and values that view the universe as a mechanical system composed of elementary material building blocks. It includes the belief that the scientific method is the only valid approach to knowledge, that life is a competitive struggle for survival, and that material progress can be achieved through unlimited technological and economic growth. These ideas are in need of radical revision. We in the church need to listen carefully to the words of Jesus:

> I thank thee, Father, Lord of heaven and earth, that thou hast hidden these things from the wise and understanding and revealed them to babes; yea, Father, for such was thy gracious will. *All things* have been delivered to me by my Father. . . . (Mt 11:25–27a)

The emergence of God's power and presence in history gives us an understanding that cannot happen in any observable, rational manner. In his scholarly work, *Encounter with God*, theologian Morton Kelsey writes:

> The direct physical effects of God's power—the healing and other manifestations or signs—were described all through the Old Testament, in nearly every book of the New Testament, and by most of the early Christian writers. Yet today it is almost impossible for us to conceive of a reality like this, existing in a world that is separate, and yet interpenetrates our own. We pass over the stories that tell of such a reality either as superstition or as the foolish ideas of uninformed men caught in an incredible world view, as myth in the "looking down one's nose" sense.
>
> If on the other hand, some men do in fact experience these powers directly, sometimes observing their visible influence in the physical world, then we are in quite a different position empirically. Then we are directly faced with the probability that there is a spiritual or nonmaterial world that does underlie the physical world and

is intimately connected with it, influencing this world in which we live in ways other than through the human psycho-physical mechanism.[4]

Kelsey vigorously challenges the conclusions of many notable theologians and philosophers, including Kierkegaard, Barth, Bultmann, Kant, Hegel, and Heidegger. Their influence, he feels, has been detrimental to a healthy spirituality that is illuminated by and emanates from Christian experience—an experience of faith that is also a praxis of faith. Kelsey has the deft ability to summarize their strengths and major weaknesses succinctly and then lead us to a fresh knowledge of God, who is always trying to break through to human consciousness. He urges us to learn to open ourselves to the divine initiative so that the Spirit can be revealed through us. We are *not* totally separated from God, and the *kerygma*—the essential message of Christ and the early church—was not somehow enveloped in an unsophisticated, premodern language of myth that conceals the truths of the gospel. Ironically, the theologians, in their attempt to be "modern," often write of God and the nature of reality within the framework of what is now an obsolete Cartesian world view. In stripping away the "myth," they have also stripped the gospel of its power. Similarly, the dispensationalists have done the same thing but for different reasons. Both have shackled the Risen Christ, mainly out of fear of appearing unscientific. Modern physics can reveal both to the reluctant theologian and to the scientist that a new world view, which allows for the numinous experience (an experience of God not rationally explainable), is in agreement with the most advanced scientific theories of reality.

Kelsey continues to challenge us regarding the reality of the Spirit:

Valid theology is built upon the converging experiences and inferences of those who have experienced numinous or religious contents. This is not much different from the way quantum mechanics has been built upon observation and inference, brought into line by going back again and again to test the actual behavior of sub-atomic particles. Theologians, thus, should be experts in religious experience, in addition to understanding the history and use of ideas and thought.

The static nature of language and its tendency towards classification tend to push us towards *either/or evaluations.* Language is full of polar opposites. Using an either/or statement tends to suggest to us that we know "all" about something. Yet the normal or statistical curve is a much better description of the way we find most things than *either/or words.* These may be valid for logic and mathematics which are not directly related to experience, but they are seldom applicable to life itself. Most of life's experiences and judgments belong to a many-point scale and cannot be squeezed into an *either/or judgment.*

Just as language has a tendency to put things together that do not belong together, it sometimes separates things which do not belong apart. Body and mind are so separated, as are time and space. Our words indicate that stupidity and intelligence, or beauty and the beast are worlds apart, but "it ain't necessarily so." Either objects or qualities may be far more closely linked than our words portray. Along with this tendency to separate things out, we also tend to look for just one cause for an event, rather than seeing that the whole field of objects forms an organic whole.

The whole problem of how things interact is very difficult to convey in ordinary language. The usual form of a transitive sentence is *actor—action—subject* [sic]. There is not the slightest hint in this grammar that the actor, too, is usually changed by his action. This is particularly true of those who think they can observe the religious experience objectively. Yet if they actually come into contact with the divine they are themselves changed. There is not even impartial observation of the smallest atom, let alone of the divine. The idea that man could be an impartial observer belonged to nineteenth-century science, and many twentieth-century theologians and philosophers are still caught in this framework.[5]

In the new physics, scientists speak of quantum theory—the theory of atomic phenomena—and relativity theory, concepts of space and time. In exploring this world they came into contact with an unexpected reality that shattered their world view and forced them to think in new ways. The new physics necessitated profound changes in concepts of space, time, matter, object, and cause and effect. Atoms consist of particles, and these particles are not made of any material "stuff." They are described as bundles of energy associated with activity and processes. They are dynamic patterns that have a space aspect and a time aspect that cannot be separated. "When we observe them we never see any substance; what we observe are dynamic patterns continually changing into one another—the continuous dance of energy."[6] Capra goes on to describe a crucial feature of quantum theory:

> The observer is not only necessary to observe the properties of an atomic phenomenon, but is necessary even to bring about these properties. My conscious decision about how to observe, say, an electron will determine the electron's properties to some extent. If I ask it a particle question, it will give me a particle answer; if I ask it a wave question, it will give me a wave answer. The electron does not *have* objective properties independent of my mind. In atomic physics the sharp Cartesian division between mind and matter, between the observer and the observed, can no longer be maintained. We can never speak about nature without, at the same time, speaking about ourselves.[7]

Our values, attitudes, beliefs, and habit patterns have a very real effect on our environment and the people with whom we come into contact. The patterns in our minds are intricately connected with the patterns observed in nature. Thus we can exert a profound influence for good or for ill.

Drawing closer to the heartbeat of God, putting on the mind of Christ, which permeates the whole of creation—"in him we live and move and have our being"—we become cocreators and colaborers in and for the kingdom. Joining forces with the Lord of movement, interaction, and transformation in the created order, we are invited into the way of healing. St. Paul admonishes us to think about "whatever is true, whatever is noble, whatever is right, whatever is pure, whatever is lovely, whatever is admirable—if anything is excellent and praiseworthy" (Phil 4:8). We are asked to fill ourselves with that which is good, because our being cannot be separated from our activity. "For as he thinketh in his heart so is he" (Prov 23:7, KJV). We, like matter, can be understood only as a whole in a dynamic context of "interconnections in an inseparable cosmic web."[8]

God's way of wholeness for the individual, through Jesus, is love. Loving our enemies, doing good to those who persecute us, turning the other cheek, walking the second mile—these are not legal obligations. They are powerful truths that transform the evil and destructiveness that would destroy life. Prayer becomes creative and meaningful, and healing is then a possibility.

But healing is considered spurious and unscientific at best in both the biological and medical sciences. Scientists continue to adhere for the most part to their reductionist models. The problems that biologists cannot solve today seem to be those which relate to the functioning of an organism as a whole, as well as its interaction with the environment. The Cartesian view of life keeps their world view narrow and fragmented. For example, only about 5 percent of DNA is used in building proteins; the rest is probably used for integrative activities about which biologists remain generally ignorant. The development of modern medicine has been integrally linked to biology, which has been dominated by a mechanistic view of life.

> The influence of the Cartesian paradigm on medical thought resulted in the so-called biomedical model, which constitutes the conceptual foundation of modern scientific medicine. The human body is regarded as a machine that can be analyzed in terms of its parts; disease is seen as the malfunctioning of biological mechanisms which are studied from the point of view of cellular and molecular biology; the doctor's role is to intervene, either physically or chemically, to correct the malfunctioning of a specific mechanism.[9]

The "problem" is corrected by an appropriate intervention such as administering a drug or performing a surgical procedure. In this way the practitioner necessarily limits herself to partial aspects of the person and achieves only a narrow view of the disorder. A person's inherent healing power (e.g., wound healing), and the instinctual drive toward health and wholeness, is rarely communicated or promoted. Life-style, living habits, and the environment are just beginning to be related to health in the traditional disease-care model. It is assumed that the doctor can repair or replace anything, even after years of abuse or neglect. This is the biomedical model that has become dogma not only for the medical profession and its institutions but also for the general public. The high technology, high cost disease-care system has become literally an idol. The hospital is the place of worship and the medical specialists are the high priests.

The same inadequate Cartesian world view that holds us bound in health keeps us dancing around the fires of economic, political, and military dominance as well. We are obsessed with winning, control, and power. In the process we trample everything and everyone who stands in our path—from the poor and dispossessed to the fragile ecosphere. Aggression at its worst, in terms of violent destructive potential, is exemplified in nuclear weapons. These "gods of metal" (Lev 19:4) are the most tragic result of people clinging to a paradigm that is no longer valid. Our choice is very clear:

> I call heaven and earth to witness against you this day, that I have set before you life and death, blessing and curse; therefore choose life, that you and your descendants may live. . . .
> (Dt 30:19)

If we are to break loose from the grip of a world view that leads us down a path of disintegration and death, we must explore a model of reality that takes into consideration the totality of man's experience, especially the Christian experience of the spiritual realm. In the following diagram, Morton Kelsey helps us visualize the possibilities.[10]

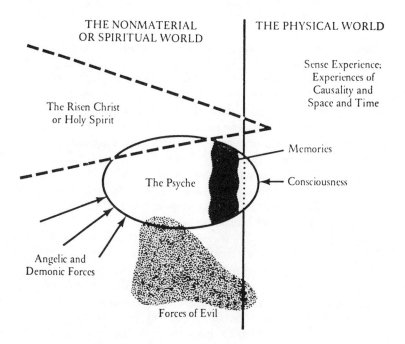

This diagram of reality agrees with the understanding of St. Augustine, who had a sophisticated view of how man reacts to both the physical and the spiritual world. He saw man as both body and spirit and capable of direct confrontation with either realm.

Again the schema represents man's relation to two worlds of experience—an outer or physical world and a spiritual one. The dividing line is purposefully shortened in the diagram. What happens beyond the limits of the line, what interactions may go on, man cannot know because he is embedded in the line between the two worlds. One can only speak about what happens within the realm of human experience. One's knowledge is of experiences and not of final things. Man seldom knows all. Whether all things are ultimately one or many is a question that has no meaningful answer; man cannot say because the answer is not experientially verifiable.

Obviously man's psyche, in his physical body, is introduced into a physical world. Through the body man has experiences of this world that at least seem purely physical, and these he relates one to another through his rational faculty.[11]

Most people, at least in the Western world, live their entire existence in a physical "box," which we can call the space-time-energy-mass continuum (STEM). We have been trained and conditioned to deny any reality that cannot be rationally quantified or measured in scientific terms according to a scientific model. Even committed people of faith who sincerely talk about life in the Spirit have real difficulty believing that there is *any* reality outside of the "box." However, the spiritual world is, in fact, the domain which encompasses that very box and gives it meaning. Even some theologians have been unable to move beyond their "boxed in" perception of reality and, therefore, the available data have not been observed. Their perception is captive within their cognitive framework, which is embedded in an obsolete world view.

As we begin to build a language to communicate our individual and common experiences, we find that God *is* encountered in our existence. God's presence in our lives is vital to our health and well-being, whether a person recognizes it or not. The new reality must break into the old one, reconciling it. Only this new reality can make us whole.

After my second year of medical school, I drove from Kansas City to California to work as a student extern in a hospital and also to spend some time with my family. I was emotionally and physically exhausted. Even though I was riding a spiritual "high" intellectually, primarily as a result of my cousin's dramatic recovery from severe mental illness, the full meaning of his healing was not yet clear to me. In fact, the event was troubling; it had turned my faith on its head and required a whole new world view to incorporate the data. (I have heard it said that it is more difficult to change someone's world view than his or her morality.) I was depressed and disgusted with medicine. Intuitively I *knew* that there was something drastically wrong—not with *what* we were learning but with the context of its application. Besides, I had been intimate to something (my friend's healing) that flew in the face of that which I was being trained to do and be. And I had just completed two years of intense, rigorous, and competitive academic medicine in the basic sciences. My class had just settled a serious dispute with the school administration, which had resulted in a two-week strike that received national media attention and had delayed final examinations. Feeling patronized and discounted during the negotiations, we students vowed to fight to the bitter end. As if this were not enough, my dad had experienced a serious heart attack during the strike and I had to fly to California.

By the end of the summer I was more rested, but I was still quite apprehensive about medicine as a career. I thought perhaps I should return to graduate studies in linguistics or enter the seminary. But intellectually I told myself that I had spent so much time, effort, and money that I "should" finish the degree program. The Lord's leading seemed unclear at best.

A running dialogue between myself and the Lord kept my mind occupied and awake during the long and tedious drive back to the Midwest. The second day I stopped early, about four o'clock in the afternoon, at a shabby motel somewhere outside Salt Lake City, Utah. I had planned to take a swim in the pool, have a light supper, go to bed early, and then get up before dawn the next morning to get a head start on the hot August day.

Sometime during the course of the night I felt a presence in my room. To know that someone is present in a room without having rational knowledge of it through our senses is not in itself a unique experience. Lying very still, I slowly opened my eyes. At the foot of my bed stood a figure of shimmering white light; it was not so bright that I could not look at it. One arm was outstretched to me. Totally without fear, I sat up in bed, reached forward, and lightly grasped the extended hand. I was immediately filled with an inexplicable sense of peace and love. I held the hand for several minutes, then went back to sleep and did not awaken again until morning. I bolted out of bed absolutely *knowing* that the figure of light was Jesus. Even as I remembered holding his hand, I knew it was the Lord. A spontaneous burst of joy and praise came forth. To this day I am certain I was awake that night and that my experience was not a dream. Not that it really matters, for as St. Paul writes, "whether in the body, or out of the body, I do not know, God knows" (2 Cor 12:2).

No words were exchanged that night, but I became aware deep within myself that my mission and ministry would spring forth from my medical training. My anxiety dissolved, and I was at peace.

My rational mind cannot explain what happened the night I encountered the One who saves and transforms. I told no one about the experience for over two years for fear of being considered unstable. But I have cherished his presence within my being.

Jesus promised to be with us always. I no longer simply believe that promise, I know it is true. For I can proclaim with Mary Magdalene, "I have seen the Lord!" (Jn 20:18).

God brings us health in many forms, but until we are touched by the reality of the Spirit, we cannot be truly whole. Our spiritual life, then, becomes a key determining factor in our journey toward wholeness. Krister Stendahl, former dean of the Harvard Divinity School, has said that God's agenda is the mending of creation. God is active in creation and is present in us—for our healing and ultimate salvation. The word *salvation*, from the root word *salvus*, means "healed." Thus, an abundant life of wholeness comes only in the mending, the healing.

St. Paul writes, "Therefore, if any one is in Christ, he is a new creation; the old has passed away, behold, the new has come" (2 Cor 5:17). Theologian Paul Tillich writes that "where there is real healing, there is this new creation, a New Being. But real healing is not where only a part of body or mind is reunited with the whole, rather where the whole itself, our whole being, our whole personality is united with itself. The New Creation is healing creation because it creates reunion with oneself. And it creates reunion with the others."[12] This is the challenge and the message of the Christian faith: healing what is fractured, giving a center to that which is estranged, and mending the rupture between God and humankind and between each other and our world. Salvation takes on a whole new perspective and meaning. "Salvation is reclaiming from the old and transferring into the New Being. This understanding includes the elements of salvation that were emphasized in other periods; it includes, above all, the fulfillment of the ultimate meaning of one's existence, but it sees this in a special perspective, that of making *salvus*, of 'healing.' "[13]

The church must again take seriously the healing ministry of Jesus and construct a world view that will give it credence and that people can truly see and hear. In order to live in a new awareness as the people of God, it is important to state and understand several assumptions:

1. God can be encountered in a real way.

2. There is a spiritual reality (including good and evil forces) that is different from, yet intimately connected to, the reality of our day-to-day existence in this world.

3. It is basically God's will that we be without sickness, that we be whole persons.

4. The triad of body/mind/spirit is one of integral interrelatedness.

5. The etiology or origin of sickness is manifold and includes physical, mental, emotional/psychological, and spiritual causes.

6. Healing occurs in many ways and is always more than a physical cure.

7. The Risen Christ can and is willing to restore health through prayer.

8. Prayer is a real source of power in achieving wholeness and promoting health, as well as in preventing and curing sickness.

9. Wellness is not in and of itself the ultimate goal.

10. Wholeness is never fully attained in this life but is an ongoing process of transformation and growth.

Healing was central to the life of the early church until about A.D. 600. The church Fathers, including Ambrose, Augustine, Gregory of Nyssa, and others, all wrote about salvation in terms of healing. There are several major causes for the decline of the healing ministry.

First, the Old Testament presents conflicting notions of a punishing/healing God. We read in Deutoronomic passages that people were sick because of God's displeasure. Deuteronomy 28:26–27 ("the Lord will smite you . . .") is seldom preached on; Deuteronomy 32:39 summarizes rather well the basic attitude of most of the Old Testament: "It is I who deal death *and* life; when I have struck it is I who *heal* (and none can deliver from my hand)." Likewise, if a person is looking for the love of God, he will not find it in this passage: "At a lodging place on the way the Lord met him and sought to kill him" (Ex 4:24). Only a Christian fundamentalist takes the entire Old Testament literally; not even the Orthodox Jew does that. The logical conclusion of this way of thinking is that if God actually sends illness and death, then it is immoral to take it away either by medical or spiritual means. However, we also see an Old Testament God of mercy who proclaims, ". . . my compassion grows warm and tender . . . for I am God not man, the Holy One in your midst, and I will not come to destroy" (Hos 11:8–9), "but with everlasting love I will have compassion on you, says the Lord, your Redeemer"(Is 54:8). This God who gives life requires only that we seek justice, love tenderly, and walk humbly *with* him (Mi 6:8).

Secondly, there *appear* to be three basic differences, which Christians have dodged with alacrity, between the Old and New Testaments. These were, however, clarified in the good news of Jesus of Nazareth who showed us the Father in himself. (1) This God, who was often seen as a vengeful Oriental monarch, Jesus called *abba*, "daddy," the one to whom we can turn to as a child turns to a loving parent. In Isaiah we are given the image of a mother with a child at breast and the promise, "I will not forget you" (Is 49:15). "He will feed his flock like a shepherd, he will gather the lambs in his arms, he will carry them in his bosom, and gently lead those that are with young" (Is 40:11). The implications are made very clear in Jesus' story of the compassionate father. The prodigal son returns to the unconditional love of his father. Jesus said that this is what the Father is like. (2) Jesus proclaimed that the kingdom of heaven is now, not just at the end of time. Therefore, the gifts of the Spirit are not only sensible but inevitable. (3) The good news is for everyone, not just the Hebrew nation. These three points clarify the whole Old Testament story. We now see a God who cares and who heals all our diseases (Ps 41:3).

The third major cause of the decline of the healing ministry is that, following the Greek perception, the church embraced a theology of reason and the five senses; there could be no contact with the nonphysical domain nor any natural intercourse between the physical and spiritual worlds. A world view in which the thinking of Aristotle and Thomas Aquinas predominated, followed in turn by Descartes, who split the body from mind/spirit, was bought in full by the church. In this kind of "box" the healing ministry must necessarily dissolve. If in this framework healing cannot stand, what must go with it? Excluding love, we lose almost fifty percent of the New Testament— revelation (including dreams and visions), discernment of spirits, gifts of wisdom and knowledge, prophecy, tongue-speaking and interpretation, the kingdom of heaven within (which can be touched). The gifts of the Spirit do not make sense; there can be no natural intercourse between God and humanity.

But God sent Jesus, the Christ, to show us that he is not far from the human condition and that we can experience the presence of the Spirit in this sinful and broken world. Kelsey points us to Christ the healer, who is the model in a new world view:

> Jesus saw it was one of his major tasks as the Christ to defeat the realities of evil that could possess men and keep them from following his way. He saw himself in conflict with the forces of evil . . . There was open warfare on a cosmic level, with physical and mental healing one of the things fought for. Failure to release man from these powers would have been unthinkable for those who saw man from Jesus' psychological point of view. And failure to heal if one had the power would have been just as unthinkable.
>
> If Jesus had any one mission, it was to bring the power and healing of God's creative, loving Spirit to bear upon the moral, mental, and physical illnesses of the people around him. It was a matter of rescuing man from a situation in which he could not help himself. Jesus disclosed a new power, a ladder to bring him out of the pit of his brokenness

and sin. Leaving man in his wretched condition so as to learn from it makes no sense in this psychological framework. Judgment and punishment only add to a burden already intolerable.

Jesus' healing actions flowed from his psychological awareness of man's nature and his experience of sonship with God . . . Unless one understands the view Jesus had of man, it is difficult if not impossible to understand the kind of fellowship he formed around him and the injunctions he gave. The New Testament does not yield a wholly clear idea of when the end of the world was expected to come, but it is very clear that the disciples were to continue in their lives to manifest as much of God's healing Spirit as they could.[14]

Living in awareness, in full reality, is ultimately revealed in the Way.

Chapter 4

Transformation, Integration, and Growth

> Do not be conformed to this world but be transformed
> by the renewal of your mind, that you may prove what
> is good and acceptable and
> perfect.
>
> *Romans 12:2*

In the struggle for wholeness, we are called to self-responsibility. The Apostle Paul exhorts us, "Work out your salvation with fear and trembling, for it is God who is at work within you . . ." (Phil 2:12–13). Salvation means more than being converted to Jesus Christ or attempting to live a sinless life or having unwavering faith. Rather, it means that our health, our wholeness, is partly a function of our willingness to be responsible for the *way* we live as the children of God. It means living within the framework of a world view in which healing is possible. The oneness of our being—body, mind and spirit—is taken seriously. We need to include in this our inherent need for healthy self-discipline and to act out of obedience, even when we don't feel like it. Positive feelings often follow the action. This in no way implies negation of God's abundant grace in our lives. Through the gift of faith we are called to be colaborers with God on the road to wholeness. It is part of proclaiming that the kingdom of God is now.

The tension lies between faithfully *resting* in the graced moments of life on the one hand and faithfully *working* to help bring forth change and growth in life on the other. St. James writes, "For as the body apart from the spirit is dead, so faith

51

apart from works is dead" (Ja 2:26). Raised in the Lutheran tradition, I have held a strong aversion to dealing with anything that even hints of "works righteousness." I know that I cannot *will* my own healing and wholeness. But I can *decide* to place my life before God so that the Spirit might work within me. I am compelled to do this continually so that I can more fully receive righteousness as a gift from God. Richard Foster writes that the spiritual disciplines

> are the *means* for receiving God's grace. God's desire is to bring us into that way of living in which our needs are cared for, our sense of identity as individuals is clarified, and the inward life becomes whole and unified. To this end, Jesus Christ lived, died, was resurrected and ever lives to be our present prophet, priest and king. The salvation that is in Christ involves not only the forgiveness of sins and heaven when we die, but the breaking of the power of sin so that we can live in newness of life now.[1]

We should add to this statement that God's desire is to bring us into that way of living in which the *outward* life becomes whole and unified as well. The dynamic tension of grace versus self-discipline is operable in the inward versus the outward journey. Integration through love becomes the fruition of both. An integrated inward life is often outwardly manifested. For example, transformation of one's mind and emotions through inner integration may become apparent in physical healing and wholeness. The causes of peptic ulcer are never cured without an inward journey and true healing. Likewise, the diseases of racism and war are rooted in inner attitudes of fear, greed, and violence. The structures of a person, family, community, society, or world must be transformed "inwardly" in order to reveal the fruits of the Spirit outwardly, according to the gifts and grace given to each. St. Paul writes in his letter to the Romans that we should present our bodies—our whole selves—to God. Then he exhorts us to seek transformation and growth through the renewal of our minds in new insights and understanding. There are many avenues to new levels of awareness. The spiritual disciplines, positive faith affirmations, and inner healing are all ways through which we can work *with* the Lord in the renewal of our minds.

In the model we began to construct in chapter 2 we saw that fear often propels us into a spiraling process downward toward disease, disintegration, and premature death. A lack of awareness leads to a lack of freedom without discipline. But the Lord invites us into a different kind of process, a different kind of freedom—one in which we seek wholeness beyond neutral living.

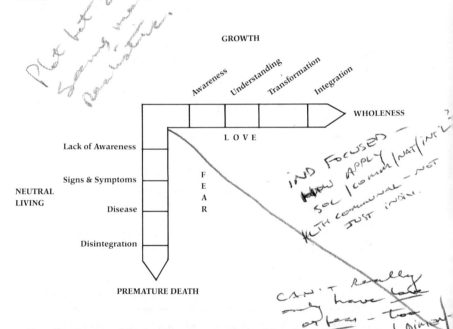

On the "neutral living" axis, motivated by fear, we deteriorate from lack of awareness, while on the "growth" axis, motivated by love, we move out from awareness through understanding and transformation to integration.

In his startling book, *The Bible in Human Transformation,* theologian Walter Wink speaks profoundly of enabling understanding through insight gained in a "wholistic" context—a movement toward transformation and growth. Wink challenges the validity of modern historical biblical criticism; he issues forth a call for a new paradigm for biblical research and study in order to render the Bible's content and meaning accessible for human development today.

> We wish to learn something from it, not better, but different, something we did not know at all, or only sensed dimly. *Respondeo etsi mutabor* (I respond though I must change): we are ready to listen even if we must change. And in rare moments of lucidity and courage we may listen *in order to change.*
>
> In order to arrive at what you do not know
> > you must go by a way which is the way of ignorance.
> In order to possess what you do not possess
> > you must go by the way of dispossession.
> In order to arrive at what you are not
> > You must go through the way in which you are not.
> And what you do not know is the only thing you
> > know. . . .
>
> This kind of knowing is not the quest for certainty about things known, but the search for the unknown. We no longer regard knowledge as a truncated pyramid in which each advance in knowledge diminishes the unknown, with an eye to its final abolition. Such an image of the intellectual quest is nothing more than an egocentric device for controlling our anxiety about existence. Instead we perceive knowledge as an inverted pyramid opening out into infinity, in which each advance in knowledge leads to greater wonder and wider vistas of unknowing. The text, the tradition, the human community, I myself—these are not problems susceptible of technological manipulation *only* (as indeed they are in the moment of agentic distance), but mysteries requiring unveiling, insight, revelation. Such knowledge is not mastery but participation received as a gift. Understanding is substituted for mastery.[2]

This is also the world view of the physicist, who in his letting go of knowing through mastery seeks the unveiling of the harmony of the universe in understanding. As Christians it is not enough for us to think of the religious experience as a final encounter that ends the need for further growth. Rather, this understanding that comes from a new awareness is the invitation into the spiritual path—the way of Jesus. Then by the gracious love of God received in human openness and trust, we are led ever deeper into the mysteries of reality toward insight, revelation, and growth.

It is painful to change, and it involves taking risks—daring to risk danger as we are called to conversion and wholeness. We cannot be transformed unless we surrender ourselves to God in every sphere of our existence: the personal, psychological, and spiritual as well as the social, economic, and political. We can then experience a change in all our relationships as we turn away from our contemporary idols. Conversion means letting God touch every part of us. The call to us is to allow God to lovingly redeem and liberate us from our worst deeply ingrained habit patterns.

It is not easy for us to move from negative thinking and speaking to positive living; our minds must be renewed. Negative thinking and negative talk produce negative results. Many of us erroneously believe that once we have expressed a negative thought it is erased from existence. That is not true. Scientific research, as well as scriptural truth, shows us that negative thinking and negative speaking produce lingering, long-term effects. Negative expressions are retained in the subconscious, and they later surface in the form of feelings, perceptions, and attitudes. A negative mindset denies the authority and power of God. A mind that is conformed to this world interprets life solely from a human viewpoint.

Many scientists in a variety of disciplines all over the world are working on composite models of the brain and mind and how they function. Our brain has at least 10 *billion* cells, and each cell has a myriad of connections. It is a marvelous and complex system, one after which we have modeled today's complex computers. The brain, together with the central nervous system, perceives and sorts out its surroundings. In the past we believed we had five senses: sight, taste, hearing, smell, and touch. But scientists now know that there are many more than five senses with which we encounter the world around us. We are bombarded with thousands, perhaps millions, of different kinds of stimuli during each second of our existence. Consider the reading of this very page: you are using your eyes. In addition, you are breathing, smelling, hearing, touching, emoting, balancing, etc. Your conscious mind conveniently sifts through and sorts out the necessary stimuli for the process of reading. Messages also reach the subconscious and unconscious parts of the mind. A great amount of information is stored there, especially unconsciously, in much the same way a computer stores information in its memory tapes.

Everything we have ever learned is recorded in the deep recesses of our brain, including the positive and the negative habit patterns. Both the good and the bad that we do come from these unconscious "tapes." For example, I see an acquaintance at church whom I am to introduce to a friend. I know the face but can't remember the name. Why? A possible explanation is that I have repetitively programed my mind: "I can never remember names, only faces." So when I ask myself the question, "What is her name?" the answer from my "computer tape" comes back immediately: "You never remember names, only faces." And so it goes with things that affect us more seriously. The computer experts have a name for this problem, GIGO— garbage in, garbage out. We need to "reprogram" or renew our minds by filling it with the good and affirming the positive.

The creative portion of the mind is the largest and most important. From a spiritual point of view, it influences our ability to receive God's power and direction in our lives. It has been estimated that even the most creative and brilliant persons, such as Einstein and Beethoven, used only about ten to twenty percent of their brain capacity. Imagine, then, what God can do in and through us if we would give God a chance!

An affirmation is a verbal description of a desired condition. We state our desire for the future in terms of the present, as if

the result had already happened. We state clearly the full out-
come that we desire, paying no attention to how it will be
achieved (that is up to God).

We have a choice when we look at the future or present. We
can consider it either positively or negatively. Some people
seem to see only the negative; they dread the future. An affirmation states that God is love and love is positive. God wants the
best for us and wants us to be joyful, whole people. Jesus said, "I
came that they may have life, and have it abundantly" (Jn
10:10). Negativity, in actuality, is elevating human judgment
over God's judgment. Those negative expressions, which are retained in the subconscious, later come forth inappropriately
and often destructively.

Our minds store thoughts, memories, and images; these can
be positive or negative. We can change negative thought patterns by inviting the Christ into those areas and asking him to
transform them through inner healing. We play a role in what
we perceive. Keith Miller writes in *The Edge of Adventure* that
when we see things through the eyes of Jesus everything
changes. When we look at things through the eyes of love, we
see less ugliness and more beauty. If we affirm and absorb God's
good will for us, we see the world differently.

We are also capable of thinking positively or negatively about
ourselves. We can think of ourselves in the past, present, or future in a positive or negative way. Faith affirmations are based
on what we know about God. Jesus, for example, is the affirmation of the Father, the very "yes" of God. A faith affirmation is
a means of verbalizing what God says in scripture as if it were
already ours in experience. Affirmations work like an electrical
circuit. If the circuit is completed, power results. If we speak
and think as God thinks and speaks about us, with love, forgiveness and affirmation, we are completing the circuit back
and forth to God. Affirmations change lives because they are an
exercise of faith that releases the power of God within a person,
and they program the subconscious mind to respond as God de-
signed it to respond.

It is important to be very specific in our "positive affirmation" because we might get something that is different from what we had expected. "I am prompt" may result in my being on time but skipping a meal or getting a speeding ticket. Maybe "I am easily on time" would better state the desired result.

Often there is no immediate result; but we need to persist, as with persistent prayer. Remember that when Jesus was asked about prayer he taught his disciples the Our Father and then immediately followed it by telling the story of the person who persistently knocked on his neighbor's door until he got the food he needed for his visitors (Lk 11:5–13). Even as the Lord wants us whole and well, we must affirm it for ourselves in actually becoming whole. If we are persistent in this positive affirmation, then God knows clearly that this is what we really desire.

Here are six ways to begin using affirmations for the renewal of our minds:

1. Write an affirmation on a piece of paper. Read it aloud over and over each evening before going to bed and the next morning when getting up.

2. Imagine or visualize yourself enjoying the desired end result as though it were happening right now.

3. Chant or sing the affirmation aloud while working, driving, playing, or praying.

4. Write the affirmation ten times in the first person: "I, Ken, can do all things through Christ who strengthens me." Then write it ten times in the second person: "You, Ken, can do all things through Christ who strengthens you." Then write it ten times in the third person: "Ken can do all things through Christ who strengthens him."

5. Record the affirmation in your own voice and listen to the recording while doing chores, driving, or going to sleep. This can be a powerful tool.

6. Choose a word, picture, or symbol. Let this symbol be a reminder of what you desire and to whom you belong—that your affirmations are in harmony with God. Put it where you will see it every day.[3]

As we are transformed in the renewing of our minds, we also

begin to be converted and liberated in other areas of our lives.
Jim Wallis warns us:

> There are no neutral zones or areas of life left untouched by
> biblical conversion. It is never solely confined to the inner
> self, religious consciousness, personal morality, intellectual
> belief, or political opinion. Conversion in Scripture was not
> a self-improvement course or a set of guidelines to help peo-
> ple progress down the same road they were already traveling.
> Conversion was not just added to the life they were already
> living. The whole of life underwent conversion in the bibli-
> cal documents. There were no exceptions, limitations, or
> restrictions.[4]

There is pain in change, and sometimes we would rather not
take the risk. It is easier to stay where we are. Abraham Maslow
writes "of the attractions of safety and security, of the functions of defense and protection against pain, fear, loss, and
threat, of the need for courage in order to grow ahead."[5]

But when we change we are actually set free. "Where the
Spirit of the Lord is, there is freedom" (2 Cor 3:17). We become
free from control by others; we are free to discover our true
selves in a balance between activity and rest; we are free to
serve others. Once the grace of God has broken into our lives
we can give up the anxiety of losing control or being controlled
by others. But these changes need integration and nurturing to
bring them together into a creative harmony.

Supported by a loving community of faith, the classical spiritual disciplines such as prayer, meditation, confession, and
worship not only lead a person deeper into a relationship with
God but also help to integrate the transformed parts of the personality. The discipline of simplicity is very important in this
life-long process of inner integration and unity. But we must be
gentle with ourselves. Growth requires patience. Seeds planted
in the fertile ground need time to germinate and take root.
Weeds also grow up alongside the good plants. In one of Jesus'
parables he warned us not to tear out the weeds lest we destroy
the plants as well. The spiritual disciplines help us to tend, to

cultivate, and to prune so that our discipleship might be pleasing to the Lord.

> Patience makes us realize that the Christian who has entered into discipleship with Jesus Christ lives not only with a new mind but also in a new time. The discipline of patience is the concentrated effort to let the new time into which we are led by Christ determine our perceptions and decisions. It is this new time that offers the opportunity and the context to be together in a compassionate way.[6]

Chronos, clock time, keeps us rushed and enslaved to our busyness. It is objective and hurried and helps fuel our fear. Clock time can be a destructive element in our model of disease, disintegration, and death.

On the other hand, *kairos*, the time of fullness and wholeness, is the time lived from within, a time of grace. It is a time when I am not afraid, a time when I can hear God's promise: "Fear not, for I have redeemed you; I have called you by name, you are mine" (Is 43:1). A physician friend of mine who is active in health ministry with the Church of the Saviour in Washington, D.C., invited a group of us, prior to a time of silent reflection, not to *do* anything, but simply to sit on the lap of God. What a beautiful image of a personal, caring Lord whom Jesus urged us to call *abba*. He bonds us to himself in love as we grow in understanding and then as we begin to help others travel that road as well. One such person the Lord brought to me was Ruth.

Ruth was a person who came to me out of deep anguish and fear. She was a well-groomed woman in her early fifties who spoke in a soft, rushed monotone, with an urgency and quality of desperation in her voice. I was moved by the story of this woman who had been suffering in the whole of her person for nearly three years. She flooded the room with a torrent of words and tears, as if she needed to say it all without interruption in fear of not being able to finish.

Ruth had lived with a disastrous marriage—a sordid relationship of alcoholism and extramarital affairs—for over twenty-five years. Her husband had been a binge drinker, and when he was drunk he became viciously cruel and abusive; she responded in kind. Somehow he had been able to hold a well-paid managerial position with a company for many years, but eventually he was fired because of his chronic alcohol problem. Together they had raised two children who no longer lived at home.

One evening while lying in bed, during one of the rare periods of relative tranquility, the television malfunctioned and caught fire. The bedroom filled with smoke and the drapes began to burn. Ruth's husband attempted to extinguish the flames with his bathrobe. His pajamas ignited and he was burned over eighty percent of his body. He died a painful death three days later in the burn unit of a local hospital.

Ruth wept bitterly as she related the vivid details of holding her husband's lifeless hand and trying to comfort his charred body during those last three horrible days. She hated him, and yet she had tried to love him in his dying. She was bitter and angry, yet she desperately sought forgiveness and reconciliation.

He died in great pain, but Ruth's pain in living was only beginning. Her adult daughter refused to attend her father's funeral; she hated her father and blamed her mother for his drinking, the ugly relationship, and for his premature death. Subsequently, both she and her brother moved out of town and refused to visit or talk with their mother.

Several days after her husband's death, Ruth began experiencing a daily recurring nightmare. She would dream of the badly burned body, from which she could not escape. Clinging to it, she was immobilized in fear and dread. She would awaken about two or three o'clock in the morning screaming hysterically, having drenched her nightgown and bed linens with sweat. This dream had occurred *every* night for three years! She could not go back to sleep, and unable to rest during the day, she was perpetually exhausted and agitated. Her very life had become a nightmare. Ruth told me that she had been treated by numerous physicians, counselors, and psychiatrists and had been put on every kind of medication without relief. She said that if something did not happen soon she was going to lose her mind or take her own life.

Ruth had quit participating in her parish, either for worship or other activities. She felt that the church could not offer any help. She had lost her religious way. She failed to follow the path of wholeness, and the community of faith did not reach out to her. Exposed to destructive forces, emotional and physical disturbances became prevalent. If sin is understood as missing the spiritual mark—*hamartia* in the Greek—then there is a very direct connection between sickness and sin. Ruth was experiencing the direct power of evil on her psyche which had observable outward effects. Jung called this direct correspondence between inner image and outer reality synchronicity.

I quietly gave thanks that she indeed had a way out and that her hope lay in the love and compassion of Jesus through inner healing. St. Peter writes, "That with the Lord one day is as a thousand years, and a thousand years as one day" (2 Pt 3:8). We can ask Jesus to walk back in time with us. We can ask him in prayer to be present at the specific moment that the hurtful event or problem occurred and to heal the painful memory. The memory remains but the pain associated with it, which can keep us in some way blocked and dysfunctional, is gone.

Recent research in the behavioral and social sciences has shown that we are profoundly affected and influenced by our environment, from the time of our conception and growth in our mother's uterus to our birth and subsequent life as infants, children, and adults.[7] The mind and body and spirit remember the love, but they also remember the hurts and the pain, even if they are no longer conscious to us. Painful memories keep us bound and can significantly affect the way we live. But in inner healing Jesus beckons to each of us, "Come to me, all who labor and are heavy-laden, and I will give you rest" (Mt 11:28). He offers himself to us, because in and through him, by his life, suffering, death, and resurrection, we are healed. We hear the promise in Isaiah:

> Surely he has borne our griefs and carried our sorrows; yet we esteemed him stricken, smitten by God, and afflicted. But he was wounded for our transgressions, he was bruised for our iniquities; upon him was the chastisement that made us whole, and with his stripes we are healed. (Is 53:4–5)

Ruth was released from her nightmares from the day we prayed together for healing. They have never returned. Ruth was able to forgive herself, her husband, and her children. She began to integrate the events of the past and to grow toward a new fullness of being and living. Through further counseling and prayer, she became reconciled with her children, began a new career, and resumed an active life in her church congregation.

Ruth's experience of encounter with a compassionate, healing God enabled her to stand against the elements that sought to destroy her. Evil and destructiveness are realities. The Apostle Paul makes it abundantly clear in his letter to the believers in Ephesus:

> For we are not contending against flesh and blood, but against the principalities, against the powers, against the world rulers of this present darkness, against the spiritual hosts of wickedness in the heavenly places. (Eph 6:12)

We are not able to handle such powers, these dark and destructive forces, on our own, but need to call upon God to come to our aid.

Ruth began to put on the "whole armor of God"—truth, righteousness, the gospel of peace, faith, salvation, and the Word of God—so that she would be able to continue to withstand and to stand. (Eph 6:13–17) She now stands as a witness in her transformation and growth to the renewing, freeing, and healing power of Jesus Christ.

It is true that we all live at different points on the coordinates of our health model at various times during our lives. We may spend a significant amount of time each day in solitude, prayer, and Christian service, but we still experience loss of self-esteem, guilt, sickness, and death. While we all must die, it will hopefully not be a premature death. As we all live, it is hopefully on the road to wholeness with its fruits of joy and peace.

The saints of the church live and die in the fullness of time; their lives can be placed to the far right on the health continuum. St. Stephen, the first martyr, died at a young age, but in wholeness. Dietrich Bonhoeffer suffered and died in a Nazi concentration camp for the sake of the kingdom. He lived in wholeness.

Sister Maria, a friend of St. Luke Health Ministries, was diagnosed as having metastatic cancer and was given only a few weeks to live. Through a combination of prayer, visualization, loving community support, and superb medical treatment, she lived more than two years and offered hope and love to dozens of people. She eventually succumbed to her disease, but she lived in wholeness.

One of my students at Johns Hopkins was helping to care for a twelve-year-old boy who had lost both his legs above the knees in an automobile accident. The child was always in good spirits, smiling and reassuring his family and the medical staff. One day the student, who was most perplexed by this seemingly inappropriate behavior, asked the boy why he was always so happy when he had lost his legs and was in pain and had to look forward to a handicapped life. The boy answered simply, "Because I know God loves me just the way I am." That is wholeness.

Love is the motivating force that propels us to wholeness. "There is no fear in love but perfect love casts out fear" (1 Jn 4:18)—God's love for us, our response to God, our love for ourselves and for others. Our experience with God is ultimately the experience of love, a love that leads from brokenness to wholeness. We love God by loving our neighbor, and we love our neighbor by doing justice. We move from domination to servanthood, from selfishness to sacrifice, from violence to peace, from oppression to liberation, from darkness to the Light of the world.

The person who is unable to let love work consciously in his life, or shuts it out because of the dangers, loses the only way man has been given to come to wholeness, integration, or healing.[8]

PART III

THE RESPONSE: HEALING AS EMPOWERER

Now to him who by the power at work
within us is able to do far more abundantly
than all that we ask or think,
to him be glory in the church and in
Christ Jesus to all generations,
for ever and ever. Amen.

Ephesians 3:20–21

Chapter 5

Living in Wholeness

May the God of peace himself sanctify you wholly; and
may your spirit and soul and body be kept sound and
blameless at the coming of our Lord Jesus Christ. He
who calls you is faithful, and he will do it.

1 Thessalonians 5:23–24

As we are healed by the unconditional loving source of all
being, transformed and integrated in Christ, we also become empowered to point the way to wholeness in and for
others. Forgiven and nurtured, we can become agents of reconciliation, healing, and peace "by the power at work within us"
(Eph 3:20). Having experienced the compassion and love of
God, we are no longer bound by fear; we are able to transcend
ourselves and enter into the suffering of others. We journey inwardly to know and experience the Risen Christ more fully; we
journey outwardly to bring God's healing presence to others.
There is an ongoing dynamic tension and balance between the
two.

Touched and changed by the power of prayer, we are called to
a life of prayer. Prayer is the key to living in graced wholeness,
empowered by the Spirit. Richard Foster writes,

> To pray is to change. Prayer is the central avenue God uses to
> transform us. If we are unwilling to change, we will abandon
> prayer as a noticeable characteristic of our lives. The closer
> we come to the heartbeat of God the more we see our need
> and the more we desire to be conformed to Christ.[1]

Prayer is a means of grace; it is a way of acknowledging the

Lordship of Jesus. It is communion with God, so that we might put on the mind of Christ (1 Cor 2:16). As Foster says, "In real prayer we begin to think God's thoughts after Him: to desire the things He desires, to love the things He loves."[2]

When we pray with the confidence that we are grafted to the Father in Jesus, we can become instruments of his healing by simply asking. "And this is the confidence which we have in him, that if we ask anything according to his will he hears us. And if we know that he hears us in whatever we ask, we know that we have obtained the requests made of him" (1 Jn 5:14–15). Since it is his will that we be whole, we can ask that he fulfill his agenda in the mending of creation. Jesus, too, invites us to ask. "Ask and you will receive, that your joy may be full" (Jn 16:24). "If you abide in me, and my words abide in you, ask whatever you will, and it shall be done for you" (Jn 15:7). Asking clearly and directly creates freedom for the one who is asked, as well as the one who is asking. David Jacobsen, in his helpful book *Clarity in Prayer* develops this theme of asking.

> The word which is translated "ask" is the Greek word *aiteo.* This word means, literally, to "crave." Now, before it is possible to crave something, it is necessary to choose that thing. To choose something, which is desired but not possessed, is to experience pain. When Jesus speaks of asking, he means choosing it and wanting it at a very deep level. It means choosing, wanting, craving. To ask or crave clearly and specifically is painful. It is also the way to get a clear answer. Unclear questions are the source of unclear responses.[3]

Questions and answers are unclear when we pray from a manipulative, bargaining, or negotiating position. But when we really surrender control in complete trust, then we can hear a clear communication of either a "yes" or a "no." In prayer God is willing to listen to us whenever we ask regardless of the position from which we come. "But our own sense of participation in the communication will be limited if we come from positions where we still control some of the response."[4] We ask our

God because we have come to love and trust; it is an act of faith to surrender control.

The quality of our question will determine the clarity of the answer. And the quality of our question is often determined by our ability to listen to *what* the Lord would have us ask, as well as to listen carefully to his response. The Latin *audire* means "to listen." This same word *audire* is also the root of our word "obedience." McNeill, Morrison, and Nouwen speak out of a depth of common experience in their profound book, *Compassion:*

> Obedience, as it is embodied in Jesus Christ, is a total listening, a giving attention with no hesitation or limitation, a being "all ears." It is an expression of the intimacy that can exist between two persons. Here the one who obeys knows without restriction the will of the one who commands and has only one all-embracing desire: to live out that will.
>
> This intimate listening is expressed beautifully when Jesus speaks of God as his Father, his beloved Father. When used by Jesus, the word *obedience* has no association with fear, but rather is the expression of his most intimate, loving relationship.[5]

Jesus obeys out of attentive listening to the loving Father. We must also learn to listen to God in prayer, especially if we seek to be God's instruments of reconciliation and healing, and seek to live in wholeness. But listening is difficult because we must move away from being the center of attention and make space for another in our inner self.

Prayer, then, is learning to communicate with our heavenly Father in asking and listening, becoming one with him and his will and empowered by the Spirit. When I invited others into my intimate space, I saw remarkable things begin to happen, and I began better to understand prayer and its connection with obedience and faith.

What was this faith of mine that had been nurtured since childhood? I remembered in James 5:15 the words, "And the prayer of faith will save the sick man." The word "save" here means "to heal" or "to make whole." And then several other scriptural verses began to make sense to me: "Now faith is the assurance of things hoped for, the conviction of things not seen" (Heb 11:1), and "Your faith might not stand in the wisdom of men, but in the power of God" (1 Cor 2:5). When I began to pray for people, I began to understand that my communion and communication with God (in asking and listening), and my daring to believe that healing could happen, was evidence of God's power and grace within me. My faith or trust became the realized hope that the Lord is risen indeed, and that by believing in faith I, and anyone else, could become God's servant—an instrument of healing.

Prayer in faith, then, becomes a means to *stand* in the power of God. The scripture provides further evidence. "For the Kingdom of God does not consist in talk, but in power" (1 Cor 4:20). "For our gospel came to you not only in word, but also in power and in the Holy Spirit with full conviction" (1 Thess 1:5). And in Ephesians we read, "Now to him who by the power at work within us is able to do far more abundantly than all that we ask or think . . ." (Eph 3:19). God can work in and through us beyond our wildest imaginations. This power or energy is what Agnes Sanford called the healing light.[6]

In recent years, researchers in physics and photobiology (the study of how light affects animals and plants) and in related fields are showing extraordinary relationships between light and health. They are convinced that all aspects of our health—mental and emotional as well as physical—are indeed affected by the intensity of light to which we are exposed, by the length of the exposure and by the color (spectral makeup) of the light.[7]

According to the latest research, light has profound effects on our immune system and may one day be used to prevent immune reactions that we don't want, such as the body's reaction to poison ivy. Light is already being used as a healing agent in a variety of physical and emotional disorders, such as depression.

We know that light is a form of energy and that all created things are made of energy. This primal, created light, which scientists are calling quarks, cannot be seen or measured; they are bursts of energy with a "tendency to exist." The physicists tell us that,

> macroscopically, the material objects around us may seem passive and inert, but when we magnify such a "dead" piece of stone or metal, we see that it is full of activity. The closer we look at it, the more alive it appears . . . Modern physics thus pictures matter not at all passive and inert but as being in continuous dancing and vibrating motion whose rhythmic patterns are determined by the molecular, atomic, and nuclear configurations.[8]

Paul advised the new Christians in Ephesus to "walk as children of light" (Eph 5:8), that is, to live as though they were made of living, moving energy such as light. Our bodies are not in fact solid matter but are made up of particles, bits of energy, that attract and repel each other with tiny explosions of light. So in a very real way the body *is* full of light.

We read in the Genesis account of creation: ". . . and the Spirit of God was moving over the face of the waters. And God said, 'Let there be light,' and there was light. And God saw that the light was good" (Gen 1:2–4). Later in the same chapter we read, "And God said, 'Let there be lights in the firmament of the heavens . . . to give light upon the earth . . . And God made the two great lights . . . he made the stars also . . . And God set them in the firmament of the heavens to give light upon the earth . . ." (Gen 1:14–17). God created light *first*, before creating the sun, moon, and stars. And that same primal living energy, God, created humankind—our very life in light. The psalmist writes, "For with thee is the fountain of life; in thy light do we see light" (Ps 36:9). This fountain of life can be tapped in prayer, so that we might receive more abundant life—an increased flow of light and energy. The creative force that made us also sustains us and dwells within our bodies, minds, and spirits. "Fear not, for I am with you" (Is 43:5). Because the Lord fills me with the energizing power of God and brings me to wholeness and health (i.e., salvation), I have nothing to fear. "The Lord is my light and my salvation; whom shall I fear? The Lord is the stronghold of my life; of whom shall I be afraid?" (Ps 27:1).

The Bible is full of expressions relating to light, to the divine illumination, to the God who is called Light. These expressions are much more than metaphors, or figures of speech; they are ways of expressing real aspects of our God. When God is called light, it expresses intimacy, for as light God cannot remain foreign to our experience.

The experience of light reveals the presence of grace infilling a person. St. Symeon of the Eastern Church states,

> We do not speak of things of which we are ignorant, but we bear witness to that which we know. For the light already shines in the darkness, in the night and in the day, in our hearts and minds. This light without change, without decline and never extinguished enlightens us; it speaks, it acts, it lives and gives life, it transforms into light those whom it illumines. God is light, and those whom He makes worthy to see Him, see Him as Light; those who receive Him, receive Him as light.[9]

The light bestowed upon Christians by the Holy Spirit is not something that comes from the outside; it appears as grace, an interior light that transforms nature. "God is called Light," says St. Gregory Palamas, "not with reference to His essence, but to His energy."[10] It is not only by analogy with physical light that God is called light. He is light insofar as he reveals himself and is able to be known. Eastern mystics in the Christian tradition would say that the divine light is given in the experience of entering into union with God. Therefore, we are speaking of reality, not allegory or abstraction.

At the moment of incarnation, "the divine light was concentrated, so to speak, in Christ, the God-man, in whom dwells the whole fullness of the Godhead bodily."[11] In the incarnation, the divine nature, totally permeated in light, joined with and deified the man Jesus. The theologians in the Orthodox tradition say that Christ during his earthly life always shone forth the divine light but that it remained invisible to most people. In a much different interpretation of the transfiguration of Jesus, the Eastern Church Fathers state that it was not a phenomenon circumscribed in space and time. "Christ underwent no change at that moment, even in His human nature, but a change occurred in the awareness of the apostles, who for a time received the power to see their Master as He was, resplendent in the eternal light of His Godhead."[12] The apostles were given a glimpse of eternal reality. To see the divine light with bodily sight, as the disciples saw it on the Mount of Transfiguration, we must participate in and be transformed by it.

Living in wholeness is opening ourselves, according to our capacity, to the divine light of God. Again, St. Gregory Palamas writes, "He who participates in the divine energy, himself becomes, to some extent, light; he is united to the light."[13] In the Gospel of St. Matthew we read, "You are the light of the world . . . Let your light so shine before men, that they may see your good works, and give glory to your Father who is in heaven" (Mt 5:14, 16). St. Paul, having been blinded by the light of the Lord on the road to Damascus, writes to the Ephesians, "Christ shall give you light" (Eph 5:14). We receive his very energy so that we might participate in the kingdom now, delivered from the powers of darkness, "to share in the inheritance of the saints in light" (Col 1:12). Jesus said, "I am the light of the world" (Jn 8:12). Jesus is the power or energy that allows us to exist. It is said that when Christ died on the cross his shed blood flowed into the earth and cleansed and energized it for all time. From the beginning of creation to its ongoing mending, "in him all things hold together" (Col 1:17).

In the field of psychoenergetics, Dr. William Tiller, a physicist at Stanford University, is opening up many new horizons.[14] He and many other scientists are exploring energy levels in the universe that are different from any we have dealt with before. These energies function differently from those that we perceive with our physical senses; we appear to have within us latent sensory systems for obtaining information at these other levels. Moreover, it appears that at some level of the universe we are all connected, as if we are part of one vast organism, just beginning to awaken and become aware of itself. Further, the generally recognized and accepted physical concepts of time, space, and matter in a three-dimensional universe are now being discovered to be mutable. That is, they can all be deformed and altered, depending on one's state of consciousness.

Einstein's relativity theory reveals the dynamic nature of matter to its fullest extent. Time becomes the fourth coordinate of the three coordinates of space to form a four-dimensional continuum. In his model of the universe, time actually slows down as speed increases and light travels in curves. Space-time diagrams have no definite direction of time attached to them. "Consequently there is no 'before' and 'after' in the process they picture, and thus no linear relation of cause and effect. All events are interconnected, but the connections are not causal in the classical sense."[15]

Our conclusion must be that whatever reality is, it is not limited to what we can perceive at the level of our physical senses. It is rather tapping into the creating, sustaining, and healing power of God, who "is able to do far more abundantly than all that we ask or think . . ." (Eph 3:20). What an exciting world we live in!

We should daily welcome the coming of the Light of the world as we allow God to infiltrate and infill our whole being. May we not only become enlightened, but empowered by the light of our Lord who overcomes all darkness!

What happens when we pray in faith with the light and power of the Holy Spirit? The sick are made whole; there is healing and forgiveness. Jesus gives us God's promise: "And whatever you ask in prayer, you will receive, if you have faith" (Mt 21:22), and ". . . Whatever you ask in prayer, believe that you receive it, and you will" (Mk 11:24). This last verse in Mark brings us back full circle to "believing in faith" and to Hebrews 11:1, "Now faith is the assurance of things hoped for, the conviction of things not seen." As an illustration, let us look at the gospel story of the healing of the woman with the hemorrhage. This woman, who had been bleeding for twelve years, was probably considered unclean and ostracized from the daily life of the community. She had spent all of her money on physicians and was no better. All she intended to do was to hide in the crowd that was pressing in around Jesus, "for she said, 'if I touch even his garments, I shall be made well' " (Mk 5:28). The bleeding stopped immediately. Yet Jesus was not content with a physical cure, and he called her forth to speak the whole truth of her life so that the healing might be complete. Only then does he say, "Daughter, your faith has made you well; go in peace, and be healed of your disease" (Mk 5:34). The woman believed in faith that she would be healed; she visualized wholeness—that which was hoped for but was not yet seen. The German poet Goethe once said, "Das was man weisst, das sieht man"—that which one *knows*, one sees. Jesus felt power go out from him. He was so in tune with the Father that, in the union of the woman's faith with his loving compassion, he was a conduit for the healing power of God. He gave her back to herself as a new creature, healed and whole. Tillich writes, "Faith means a power that shakes us and turns us, and transforms us and heals us. Surrender to this power is faith."[16]

Prayer itself is an act of faith, and through faith we are empowered. In that power is the kingdom of God—the power of the Holy Spirit—to effect real healing of a person individually, in relationships with others, and in the world.

There are, however, blocks to healing and many reasons why people are not healed and do not experience wholeness in this life. Francis MacNutt articulates these well in his books *Healing* and *Power to Heal*. To help overcome these blocks I would like to propose some guidelines, in a format of eight steps, that I believe are very useful in prayer for healing. They are not meant to be rigid rules, only gentle reminders. Many people have found them helpful as they themselves are embraced by our healing Lord and then begin reaching out to others in prayer and compassionate solidarity.

1. *Praise.* As St. James says, "Let him sing praise" (Ja 5:13). Give praise to God for his mercy and goodness, that he loves us, cares for us, and heals us. We are urged to "offer the sacrifice of

praise to God continually, that is the fruit of our lips, giving thanks to his name" (Heb 13:15). Praise brings us into worship, before the throne of grace, so that we can experience the reality of the Risen Christ in our midst and be filled with the joy of the Lord.

2. *Guidance or Discernment.* We have been promised that the power of the Spirit of Jesus is with us. It is important to ask for guidance to help discern the reasons for praying. Perhaps a physical problem is really a manifestation of emotional turmoil and prayer for inner healing is needed. Learn to listen with one ear to God and the other to the person for whom you are praying. St. James writes, "Draw near to God and he will draw near to you" (Ja 4:8). But remember also his admonition, "You ask, and do not receive, because you ask wrongly" (Ja 4:3). The prayer for guidance constantly surrounds the prayer of faith.

3. *Belief.* After asking for guidance, we must believe, trusting in God that something will really happen. "And whatever you ask in prayer, you will receive, if you have faith" (Mt 21:22). We pray also that the gift of faith might be increased in us so that we might be empowered to "move mountains" (Mt 21:21).

4. *Forgiveness.* Confession and forgiveness are realities that transform us, individually and corporately. "Confess your sins to one another, and pray for one another that you may be healed" (Ja 5:16). Foster reminds us that "the followers of Jesus Christ have been given the authority to receive the confession of sin and to forgive it in His name."[17] The words of St. John speak clearly: "If you forgive the sins of any, they are forgiven, if you retain the sins of any, they are retained" (Jn 20:23), and "If we confess our sins, he is faithful and just, and will forgive our sins and cleanse us from all unrighteousness" (1 Jn 1:9). Unforgiveness is often a block to healing.

5. *Anointing with oil.* Anointing the forehead of someone with oil in the sign of the cross and in the name of the Lord (Ja 5:14) is an ancient tradition in the church. It connects us to our baptism and serves as a sacramental sign in healing. Historically, oil was thought to have medicinal value and is referred to

in the Talmud. Today we can think of it as a powerful symbol of God's healing—present not only in prayer but in all the healing and medical arts and sciences.

6. *Touch.* Touching a person imparts not only human warmth, love, and compassion psychologically but actually transfers energy as well. What we theologically can call divine light or the healing light, modern scientific research is showing to be true.[18] Jesus, our model, touched people who needed and sought healing. "Now when the sun was setting, all those who had any that were sick with various diseases brought them to him; and he laid his hands on every one of them and healed them" (Lk 4:40). Jesus touched even lepers, which was unheard of in his culture. In Matthew 8:3, a leper asks if Jesus would be willing to heal him. "And he stretched out his hand and touched him saying, 'I am willing; be cleansed.' " Jesus makes a profound statement about the love of the Father in touching even the most revolting person in the eyes of that society. The disciples learned from the Master, and they touched people. We, too, are asked to become channels of God's healing power in this way.

7. *Visualization.* God sees us whole, made in his image. So, too, we should visualize the same wholeness and healing that God intends for the person for whom we are praying. The mind has the wonderful ability to summon and hold certain images. Our emotions and physiology are likely to follow the direction set by our mind. Despite the fact that the link between visualization (imaging) and neurophysiological alteration remains an enigma, there is increasing evidence that subtle mental phenomena can have a profound positive or negative impact upon an individual's entire psychophysiology. By praying as specifically as possible, visualizing a positive image of health (whether an organ, an emotional response, or the total person), we *affirm* the power of God and *deny* power to any negative image. The Apostle Paul declares, "And we all, with unveiled faces, reflecting the glory of the Lord, are being changed into his likeness from one degree of glory to another . . ." (2 Cor 3:18).

8. *Thanksgiving.* End the prayer with thanks to God that

what you have asked for in faith shall indeed be so. In gratitude that God has heard us, we exclaim with the psalmist, "We give thanks to thee, O God; we give thanks; we call on thy name and recount thy wondrous deeds" (Ps 75:1).

> Bless the Lord, O my soul; and all that is within me, bless his holy name! Bless the Lord, O my soul, and forget not all his benefits, who forgives all your iniquity, who heals all your diseases, who redeems your life from the Pit, who crowns you with steadfast love and mercy, who satisfies you with good as long as you live so that your youth is renewed like the eagle's. (Ps 103:1–5)

As faith is a prerequisite, so love is the heart of prayer for healing and reconciliation. The community of faith and love serves the Lord by reaching out to others in love. It is the sign of the kingdom of God. "By this all men will know that you are my disciples, if you have love for one another" (Jn 13:35).

Healing is more than an individual event. The people of God are called to be a healing and praying community. As a living witness to a life of wholeness—spiritually, physically, mentally, socially, economically, and politically—we are to pray for peace, the earth, the poor, justice, and an end to violence everywhere. We must eagerly seek the values of the kingdom of God, the values Jesus lived and taught. We of the St. Luke community know that in order for healing to be complete, families, communities, whole nations, and the structures of society as well as individuals must be reconciled. We join in affirming this with the Sojourners community in Washington, D.C.; they live as a powerful witness for the contemporary church. Jim Wallis, founder and pastor, makes it poignantly clear:

> The kingdom indeed represents a radical reversal for us. Aggrandizement, ambition, and aggression are normal to us and to our society. Money is the measure of respect and power is the way to success. Competition is the character of most of our relationships, and violence is regularly sanctioned by our culture as the final means to solve our deepest conflicts. The scriptural advice "Be not anxious" challenges

the heart of our narcissistic culture, which, in fact, is anxious over everything. To put it mildly, the Sermon on the Mount offers a way of life contrary to what we are accustomed. It overturns our assumptions of what is normal, reasonable, and responsible. To put it more bluntly, the Sermon stands our values on their heads.[19]

The values, attitudes, and activities in a mechanistic, Cartesian world view, which include obsession with "hard" technology and science and an overemphasis on material acquisition and expansion, have institutionalized greed, pride, and selfishness—even in the church.

But Jesus calls blessed those who live in a way radically different from that which our society espouses. As we hear the call to wholeness, the spiritual disciplines become central to growth through transformation—to growth in the life of the Spirit.

Prayer for the healing of the nations is as vital as prayer for the healing of persons. Both are interconnected and interdependent, and the same steps that have been discussed above can and should be applied. In both we need to start by acknowledging our utter dependence upon God and praying that by his grace we might share in his love and mercy. Wallis strikes the clarion call for communities of faith:

> The greatest need in our time is not simply for *kerygma*, the preaching of the gospel; nor for *diakonia*, service on behalf of justice; nor for *charisma*, the experience of the Spirit's gifts; nor even for *propheteia*, the challenging of the king. The greatest need of our time is for *koinonia*, the call simply to be the church, to love one another, and to offer our lives for the sake of the world. The creation of living, breathing, loving communities of faith at the local church level is the foundation of all other answers. The community of faith incarnates a whole new order, offers a visible and concrete alternative, and issues a basic challenge to the world as it is. The church must be called to be the church, to rebuild the kind of community that gives substance to the claims of faith.[20]

That substance is made manifest in the word compassion. When we hear the word compassion, it generally evokes a positive response in us. We think of helping someone, showing love, and expressing sympathy or empathy. We like to think of ourselves as possessing those qualities of compassion that make us "feel good" or "warm" inside. However, a closer look at compassion reveals a depth of meaning that we may not be willing to consider. The roots are from the Latin *cum* and *pati*, meaning "to suffer with." "Wait a minute," we protest. We are willing to offer loving gestures by providing dry goods for the church food pantry, or visiting a hospitalized neighbor, or praying for a friend's imprisoned nephew. But suffering is something we can do without. It is something we most often want to avoid at all costs. Considered in this way, compassion takes on negative overtones for many people.

But compassion is not simply a sentimental feeling or concept. It lies at the very heart of gospel servanthood. Compassion means letting go of our pride, our competitive striving selves, and the defenses that wall us off from our brothers and sisters. It means that we are willing to be patient and vulnerable, to risk getting hurt. Compassion allows us to open up a space to another in our innermost being and really to listen and hear that person in his/her brokenness and pain. If we truly believe that God is real and can be encountered, if God is with us—in and among us—then we have no reason to be fearful. Because the kingdom is now, the Lord is reigning. And because God is reigning, we can live in freedom and wholeness. But we must be willing to dare to risk taking Jesus at his word, that he is with us always.

In faith through God's grace we are called to a life of love, which impels us to compassionate discipleship in prayer and service. To be compassionate means to reach down into the pain of another, to stand in solidarity and to suffer with that person. It means loving the suffering person, the one in pain, fully and completely like the Father in Christ who loves. Love is the motivating and initiating force toward health, healing, and wholeness. Jesus admonished us to "be compassionate as your Father in heaven is compassionate." If the Father's agenda is the mending of creation, then it is in loving compassion (God's love for us, our love for self and others) that healing can take place, that wholeness can be restored.

Helping to stock the food pantry in a suburban church can be a very "removed" act of charity. Serving the hungry and homeless in a soup kitchen in the inner city may be our call to compassion and servanthood. In praying for God's healing presence with a neighbor or friend we become more compassionately present and vulnerable than if we simply sent flowers or chatted at the bedside. In working with women or men in prison we begin to see reflected our own secret and inner pain, anger, jealousy, lusts, and greed. We begin to move in compassion from judgment to seeking justice, from disintegration to transformation and growth, from fear to love in Jesus' name.

Prayer is the way of the compassionate life. Real prayer is empowering change. It is risky business to let God into our lives. When we touch the heartbeat of God in prayer, we experience the One who saves and transforms. Although the cost of discipleship may be high, we can serve authentically and bring healing to the woundedness of those in need in our families and communities. Compassion is an integral part of the call to wholeness.

Far more than we realize, our very presence has an impact on the people and world around us. The glimpses of reality provided by the subatomic physicists in their inspired search for truth and the presence of the Spirit in our lives show us that there is no reality apart from our observations, evaluations, and judgments about it. If an observer's or participant's energy field interacts with, and thus changes, the energy field of the whole system, then how much more powerful the effect when that energy is channeled in prayer. We are more than bystanders; we have a definite part in structuring our own lives and the lives of others. Gathered in prayer as an Easter people,[21] we are truly colaborers with God as we help to create a reality of healing, reconciliation, and wholeness.

Chapter 6

Caring for the Whole Person

> Blessed be the God and Father of our Lord Jesus Christ,
> the Father of mercies and God of all comfort, who com-
> forts us in all our affliction, so that we may be able to
> comfort those who are in any affliction, with the com-
> fort with which we ourselves are comforted by God.
> *2 Corinthians 1:3–4*

I was surprised and delighted to meet Marina at a neighborhood birthday party. I had not seen or talked with her
for almost a year. She had been one of my favorite students at
the university, and she was in the midst of doctoral studies in
international health. I had been her adviser in the development
of a research project.

Marina spoke English fluently with a strong Spanish accent,
which revealed her roots in Latin America. She was articulate,
very bright, and wanted to do something significant in health
care to help her people. I was pleased to see her, and I was anxious to hear how her research was progressing.

We began our conversation with the customary social pleas-
antries, but when I remarked on the amount of weight she had
lost, Marina's expression darkened. Lightly touching my arm
and lowering her voice, she whispered, "Dr. Bakken, I have a
problem. I have been told that I have anorexia nervosa. I'm not
eating, and when I do eat, I vomit soon after the meal. Please,
can we talk?"

Sinking into a chair in one corner of the dining room, I wondered at her immediate candidness, and yet I was grateful for

her trust in me. "What's happened to you?" I proceeded cautiously, following my intuition that now was a good time to hear her story.

"Since I last talked with you, I had to change my doctoral research due to the sensitivities of the political situation at home," Marina began. She indicated that she was happy about her new project, and yet I was keenly aware of the excitement and intense energy that she had expended on the first one. Marina promised me that she would one day complete it.

"I have a boyfriend now—my first one, really—with whom I am deeply involved. I love him very much, but I don't think he has the same commitment to me.

"Something happened between us last fall. I stopped eating. I couldn't eat. I went back home, back to my country, for a few weeks to visit my parents. I thought I would feel better. But I ate only a few meals the whole time I was there, and I vomited after each of them. I became so sick that I was admitted to the hospital for a few days. I was seen daily by a psychiatrist and she diagnosed my problem.

"When I returned to Baltimore I still did not eat, and when I tried, I always vomited. Actually, I am happy about it, because I am losing a lot of weight. I've lost over forty pounds in the past two and one-half months. I have been fat all my life and now I want to be thin. What's wrong with that?"

I was somewhat startled by Marina's sudden intensity and defensiveness because I had been listening without comment. I replied, "Nothing. It depends on how you lose it and what you think about yourself. What did the psychiatrist say?"

"I have a bad image of my body from the neck down." I suppressed a spontaneous chortle by pretending to cough. "She said I have to learn to accept myself and deal with my relationship with John."

This was not the same Marina I had known at the university—an intelligent young woman with a *joie de vivre* and boundless energy. She was obviously depressed, and life was out of control. I felt a deep sense of compassion for Marina, and I wanted her to know that I cared. But the laughing sounds of the party celebration heightened; it was an awkward place and time to share much more. I explained briefly to her our work at St. Luke's, and I asked her if she would please come to see me soon at the health center. She promised to call for an appointment after the Christmas holidays.

Sitting in my office three weeks later, Marina quietly reviewed for us (our health assessment team of physician, nurse educator, and pastoral counselor) what she had told me at the party. She had seen her psychiatrist during the Christmas break at home and had gotten a few new insights, which she willingly shared. But she ended by saying, "I am no better and still have not eaten. I am losing hope." I detected a deep sadness and resignation in her voice.

Marina's boyfriend claimed to love her, but the previous fall, just before Marina became ill, he had become involved with another young woman who lived in the same apartment building. He had expressed his reliance on Marina to nurture his emotional and intellectual needs, and he claimed that the other relationship provided primarily sexual gratification. Marina had maintained her virginity even to the point of refusing to kiss him, while at the same time permitting and encouraging heavy petting. She had insisted on a mutual commitment to eventual marriage, which John was unable to make, before she would even consider kissing or sexual intercourse. Marina stated that she did not want to lose John; she also did not want to violate her moral standards. She refused initially to acknowledge her growing anger at his dependency upon her while exploiting the favors of another woman. The session concluded with a short prayer in which we asked the Lord to reveal to Marina the real root of her eating disorder.

During the second session the following week, Marina began to verbalize that she thought withholding food from herself was probably an unconscious way to punish John. She then began to express her hurt and anger at his behavior, whereas previously she had wanted only to explain it away and excuse him. It became clear to Marina that she had avoided the issues that had kept her obese and which now threatened to overwhelm and destroy her: lack of self-esteem and self-acceptance, and a love relationship with a confusion about its sexual/genital expression. Here was a turning point, a paradigm shift to be grasped, a recognition of the problem, as well as insight into the opportunities that now seemed possible. Gathered around Marina in prayer, we asked God very specifically to fill her with light and life, to heal her.

On the third visit Marina appeared relaxed and radiant; I had not seen her this way since she was in my class. It took some coaxing for her to share with us the significant event that had transpired that week.

"I don't think I am one of those people, am I?" Marina asked.

"What people?" I questioned.

"People who are visited," she responded hesitantly. "Last Tuesday after I left here, I went home. I was lying on my bed and the most amazing thing happened. I don't know whether I was awake or dreaming or imagining it or what." There was excitement in her voice, which began to resonate with the intuitive stirrings within me.

"I saw a large ball of bright light hovering over my bed. It came closer and closer until it covered me and became one with me. The next thing I remember I was floating and looking at myself as I lay on the bed, very still and unafraid. Then it all ended as quickly as it had begun. I got up, feeling incredibly peaceful and quiet. And then I knew that it was over. Everything was OK. I prepared a salad for myself and I have eaten every day since. I know that I am well now."

My eyes welled up with tears at the remembrance of the Light of the world who had filled me with grace and peace nearly ten years before. "You are truly blessed. The Lord has touched you, Marina."

Marina is fully recovered. She has worked through her poor self-image and her relationship with John. Transformed by the Spirit of God, the broken parts have now been integrated into the whole. She is completing her doctoral dissertation, teaching part time, and living, by the grace of God, a full, joy-filled, rewarding life.

In caring for Marina as a whole person, we were for her the church, a healing community. Indeed, our contemporary quest for health and wholeness must begin in the church and its congregations. The vocation to serve as a healing community has its origin in the life and teachings of Christ. Health in its fullest meaning must no longer be abdicated to those who continue to propound an obsolete world view. In *A Study of the Healing Church and Its Ministry: The Health Care Apostolate*, prepared for the Lutheran Church in America in 1982, Ralph Peterson challenges us to remember who we are.

> The recovery of the missionary mandate to health care calls us to recover the Resurrection Life that is ours in the Body of Christ. The call to health care demands a converted church, a church that is healed by the power of the Spirit. Our problem is not that we don't have services of faith healing. Our problem is that we do not live in apostolic faith and experience the healing and hope that come from being an Easter people.[1]

The church has always been involved in innumerable practical actions to treat sickness. Especially since the time of the reformers, Christians have established hospitals, clinics, and medical schools wherever missionary groups have gone. But "by a strange quirk of logic it is permissible to remove medically the results of man's sins, but it is not quite correct to believe God will do it himself if asked in prayer or invoked through sacraments."[2]

The church has tried, most often schizophrenically, to maintain a Cartesian world view and still claim the ultimate power of God as creator, healer, and sustainer. God becomes either a whimsical cosmic bellhop—a notion that only a weak, if not heretical, theology can support—or is put into a box on the shelf to be protected by "liberal" or "fundamentalist" doubletalk. Christian health practitioners have brought the loving model of Jesus to their work of treating sickness, but generally they are limited by the dogmatic stance of the biomedical model that reduces health to mechanical functioning. They have been unable to deal with the phenomenon of healing satisfactorily. Capra makes it clear that this is the most serious shortcoming of the biomedical approach.

> Although every practicing physician knows that healing is
> an essential aspect of all medicine, the phenomenon is con-
> sidered outside the scientific framework; the term "healer"
> is viewed with suspicion, and the concepts of health and
> healing are generally not discussed in medical schools.[3]

Only recently are these concepts beginning to be discussed in
the church in earnest. We are now beginning to realize that the
functions that are crucial to our health and well-being—
integrative activities and interactions with the environment
—do not lend themselves to a reductionist description. By con-
centrating on smaller and smaller fragments of the body, we
have not been able to cure, or even to understand, most of today's prevalent diseases and problems. A whole-person,
ecological-systems approach is needed. For as Capra explains:

> Systems theory looks at the world in terms of the inter-
> relatedness and inter-dependence of all phenomena, and in
> this framework an integrated whole whose properties can-
> not be reduced to those of its parts is called a system. Living
> organisms, societies, and ecosystems are all systems.[4]

Healing is possible, in modern scientific terms, when an integrated organism generates a coordinated response to distressful
environmental influences. This implies concepts and approaches that transcend the Cartesian split. For the Christian,
it implies the transforming and integrating presence of the One
in whom "we live and move and have our being" (Acts 17:27).

The commitment of the St. Luke Health Ministries has
been to develop and implement creative ways to empower
communities of faith in healing. We are attempting to stimulate, enlarge, and temper the curative care/crisis orientation
approach that now prevails. By setting our contemporary obsession with treating illness into the larger framework of
health care and the meaning of wholeness, we are beginning
to synthesize the ecological sensitivities of: (1) personal and
corporate responsibility, (2) spiritual and emotional growth,
(3) health promotion and disease prevention, and (4) social

and political activism. Healing, in fact, falls properly under the rubric of liberation theology. "For the kingdom of God means liberation from the powers of death, freedom from the powers that squelch life—whether through war, social injustice or physical illness."[5] The gospel proclaims life, freedom, and love. Liberation comes in recovering that which the oppressor—in whatever form of evil—has taken. Liberation is always connected with the experience of God. It is the reign of justice and wholeness.

St. Luke's is a growing ecumenical community of believers for whom health has become a vehicle for renewal in the church. The staff is comprised of a variety of health professionals, including physicians, clergy, religious, nurses, and counselors, all of whom are dedicated to prayer, service, and a life immersed in the gospel imperatives. Our greatest strength, however, lies with the many St. Luke volunteers, both professional and lay, who are "able to comfort those who are in any affliction" (1 Cor 1:4). We believe that our health community is, in the first instance, a sacrament of Christ; we represent him, re-present him, make him truly present. We struggle to become a sign, a prolongation of the healing Lord.

There are several key components to the framework that we are developing.

1. *Whole person health care* at the St. Luke Health Center addresses the physical, emotional, and spiritual aspects of those who come for care. The approach is based on a model developed by Granger Westberg: underutilized church space is converted into a modern health-care facility and is staffed by an interdisciplinary team of physician, nurse, and pastoral counselor. James Gordon writes that these team members

> are concerned with helping their patients heal the split that has stripped the mind of its power to experience and control the body, that has stripped the body of its wisdom and intentionality, and has ruptured the bond between these two and the spirit that gives them both meaning.[6]

We call patients "participants" because we believe that we

are all coparticipants in health, each one seeking his or her own way to wholeness. The practitioner is a participant on the path to healing. Because the uniqueness of each person is emphasized, enough time must be spent with the person to enhance understanding of the complex socio-economic, biological, genetic, psychological, and spiritual factors that characterize his or her illness or health. People must be considered in the context of their culture, their family, and their community if they are to understand how they experience life. Theoretically, this also helps to incorporate other significant persons into the therapeutic process.

Participants are encouraged to take responsibility for their health, which includes learning techniques that rely primarily on their own efforts rather than the practitioner's. Practiced daily, progressive relaxation linked with prayer and meditation can be an important tool for a person who is chronically anxious and tense. Emphasis is placed on innovative approaches that promote behavior patterns that will improve one's health status, sense of well-being, and longevity. But individuals do have a choice. They can perpetuate poor health habits, such as smoking and overeating, that can result in a lowered quality of life, disease, and premature death, or they may make changes that will reduce risk factors, mobilize their innate capacity for self-healing, and improve their overall health.

The setting of the health center is also very important. St. Luke's is an intimate place that encourages personal interaction between participants and staff. Our presence in a church is a powerful symbol, as are the many other symbols within the health center, which are constant reminders that our faith in the resurrected and living Lord is central to all that we do. There are several modern clinic and counseling rooms, but the most important place in the center is the prayer room. Carpeting, a few large pillows, a Bible, a candle, a potted plant, and a cross fashioned from the rough-hewn logs of a dogwood tree give it a warm and simple "feel." This quiet place of prayer witnesses to our belief that the Christ is the source of all health. Every participant is offered the gift of prayer.

The health center is located in a racially integrated, lower middle-class neighborhood situated in the midst of poverty and bordered by a more affluent area. Many different kinds of people from all walks of life seek our help. But in radical obedience to Jesus Christ, we feel called to identify with the poor and oppressed. His gospel was preached to the poor; the powerless, the vulnerable, the hurting, the weak, the defenseless flocked to hear him and be healed by him. He chose to serve them. "If the poor were Christ's people and we are his body, then the poor become our people. If Christ was the servant of the poor, then, among the poor, the church lives as a servant people."[7] Jesus' teaching is the pattern for our discipleship. No one is turned away for lack of financial resources. We have feared that we might fail financially. There are thousands of discounted, powerless people who are not covered by Medicare or Medicaid programs and who have "fallen between the cracks." For these people monetary reimbursement is not possible. But we have begun slowly to trust the Lord's generosity. He provides for our needs, our "daily bread."

Although there may be the occasional necessity for swift and authoritative medical or surgical intervention, the emphasis at the health center is on helping participants to understand and to help themselves, on education and self-care rather than on treatment and dependence. As a staff, we see ourselves as resources and facilitators rather than as parental-like authorities. Our job is to share knowledge rather than to mystify and withhold it. Each team member carefully observes the person and situation, describes and records the encounter in spiritual as well as traditional clinical terms, integrates and synthesizes the information, and then shares it with the participant. Together, or in conference with other staff members, they develop a plan of action, whether a curative intervention or a change in lifelong habits, to restore and promote health. Participants are listened to, touched, and hugged; we cry, laugh, and pray with them. They are encouraged to explore their bodies and their minds and to seek the Spirit who pervades it all. Jesus declared, "I came that they might have life, and have it abundantly" (Jn 10:10).

Joan came to the health center seeking help for her insomnia, depression, and overweight. She had recently been divorced from her husband and was unable to find a job. As a physician, I was the first staff person to see Joan. She requested medication for her depression, which she said would also help her sleep; she had received it before from another doctor. After a thorough examination, I gently suggested that we begin to explore in greater depth the *reasons* for her problems, rather than mask the symptoms with a drug, and hope that they would eventually disappear. She agreed somewhat reluctantly. I requested that before the next appointment she write down those things that she felt held her bound—those things that remained locked up and unforgiven deep within her. In her journal she shared her pain.

> I cannot be open with people I love because I do not like the person (myself) that would be exposed. I lie to protect a good self-image when I really am a foolish and vain person. I cannot express my anger because I do not trust my feelings. I cannot risk being angry and causing a person to reject me because of that anger. I fear being out of control and not knowing what I may say or do.

Herein lay the essence of Joan's depression and insomnia. With the pain articulated and acknowledged, we could begin to help her, through counseling and prayer for inner healing, to accept herself and God's unconditional love for her. The intense feelings of guilt and anger were released. Dietary and exercise counseling with a nurse helped Joan lose weight and gain a new appreciation of her body. She began to experience joy and peace—gifts of the healing Spirit—for the first time in many years. What was touched in her existential reality was a *whole* woman—not just an angry, disordered personality or an obese abdomen (although they both were part of her).

2. *Home Health Ministry* is an important component in mobilizing the community of faith in caring for their own health and that of their neighbors. Outreach into the home, especially for the frail elderly, homebound, and handicapped, provides a source of support that complements a health center

ministry. The traditional commitment of the church to the welfare of the sick and infirm provides a strong basis for collaboration in organizing and delivering volunteer-care services.

There are more than 10 million health-impaired Americans who experience difficulty in performing without assistance such essential daily activities as feeding, bathing, and dressing. Approximately one-half of these individuals are elderly, for whom institutionalization can be avoided if they receive support for their personal care. Many are poor and do not have the financial resources to pay for any kind of home care, especially when the informal networks of family and friends break down. A nursing home can be an unsatisfactory alternative because institutionalization of an impaired person often hastens a decline in health.

The primary goal of the outreach program of St. Luke Health Ministries has been to increase the abilities of elderly, disabled, and other needy people to live in their own homes with maximum health and personal satisfaction. To accomplish that end, the major emphasis has been to help church volunteers support their members and persons in the surrounding community who are frail, ill, isolated or who have other health or social needs. It is to call the people of God to renewed action in the compassion of Christ. Jesus tells us that he came into the world not to be served but to serve, and so it is with us. We need to listen again to the words of our Lord after washing the feet of his disciples: "For I have given you an example, that you also should do as I have done to you" (Jn 13:15). My colleague once said to me, "Ken, when I am in one of these homes, in some real way I feel as if I am serving Jesus himself." He had experienced one of the wonderful mysteries of the faith and the full import of Jesus' words: "Truly I say to you, as you did it to one of the least of these my brethren you did it to me" (Mt 25:40).

It is scandalous that the Body of Christ is divided and fragmented. When we focus on that which unites us rather than on that which divides us, the power of God can flow forth in new and enriching ways. Congregations representing seven major denominations have formed an ecumenical coalition for health and healing ministry in the St. Luke target area. The intention of the Health Ministry Council is to enhance and utilize the invaluable resources of faith, love, and good will of Christ-inspired congregations to support, encourage, serve, and pray for their members and neighbors in need. St. Luke Health Ministries provides resources for education, training, supervision, and consultation to the Council and member churches. Training programs are conducted for Health Promoter volunteers from each congregation who learn practical skills and knowledge for physical, emotional, social, and spiritual support of their church community.

Parishes are encouraged to organize a Health Ministry Committee if such a group does not already exist. Such a committee, in collaboration with the professional staff and lay leadership of the church, would develop a roster of active and inactive members and friends who are chronically ill, disabled, or socially isolated. Lists of neighbors or others without formal church associations would also be drawn up and efforts made to discover and enhance informal ties with those living in the neighborhood. Responsibility for these nonmembers is shared by member churches of the larger Health Ministry Council. Health ministry committees in each congregation are encouraged to establish regular visitation schedules as well as a telephone contact system.

As we begin to live and act as an interconnected and interdependent people, once again the world will say of Jesus' followers, "See how they love one another." We must be the visible form of invisible grace.

3. *Local churches* in which a Health Ministry Committee or its equivalent is part of the official structure often experience a deepening commitment to renewal of healing within the parish. The community of faith has been an unrecognized and untapped resource in health. Only recently has it begun to realize its potential to lead people to new levels of aware and responsible healthful living.

The Health Ministry Committee serves both as an umbrella and as a catalyst. It helps to clarify the many healing activities that are already happening in most churches—prayer groups, worship, baptism, the Eucharist, visitation, fellowship dinners, hymn sings—and to stimulate new awarenesses and activities. Each congregation is encouraged to have a special health-emphasis week every year that includes seminars, conferences, worship services, and celebrations to heighten the knowledge and reality of healing and wholeness. One large parish celebrated the Festival of St. Luke for three days in October with a free community health fair, healing service, guest speakers and workshops on such topics as stress control, healing in the parish, new paradigms in health, and experiential programs in relaxation, exercise, and spirituality.

The Eucharist is a service of healing *par excellence.* The Lord himself invites us to his table to partake of his very being, to become one with him. Morton Kelsey reminds us that he who offered his life for us offers us wholeness through his body and blood.

> The great value of Christianity is that it is the most materialistic of all religions; it emphasizes the spirit, but within the framework of the material world. Christianity is never one-sided or unbalanced when it follows Jesus of Nazareth. Its central message is that God became man, that spirituality indwelt the flesh and the two realms came together. This continues to be expressed in the central service of Christianity, the eucharist or communion service, in which the bread—from the grain grown by the sweat of man's toil in the fertile, dark earth—and wine—pressed from the fruit of the green vine—are made carriers of the very powers of spirituality.[8]

The power to be made whole is expressed in the liturgical response: "Lord, I am not worthy to receive you, but only say the word and I shall be healed." The Christian community needs to gain a new sense of appreciation for this healing gift that our Lord has freely given us.

One sign of renewal the Spirit of God is evoking in the church has been the institution of services of prayer for healing. One might ask, "Why do we need a healing service when we have communion and prayer groups?" The reason is simple yet profound: a special healing liturgy is a powerful symbol of obedient response to the Lord's command to heal the sick. It makes visible and explicit what the church for too long has failed to proclaim—that Christ's encounter with us is healing and that the kingdom of God is now.

It is the experience of St. Luke Health Ministries that prayer for healing in the church is best introduced after careful preparation of the congregation. An adult-seminar series on Sunday mornings or during the week covering topics of world view, historical, philosophical, and theological perspectives of health, healing, and prayer are vital to successful implementation. Otherwise, the backlash due to ignorance, misunderstanding, and fear may squelch the best intentions of a pastor and the lay leadership. St. Luke's began working with a large congregation in which a prominent member, who also had been the architect of their beautiful sanctuary, stated emphatically that the day there was "faith healing" in his church would be the day he walked out. A well-planned, rather scholarly ten-week Lenten seminar series in which the St. Luke staff participated was attended by forty to fifty persons on Sunday mornings. The series culminated with a very moving healing service at which over 100 people were present. It seems that in this congregation no one is now opposed to the newly formed Health Ministry Committee and the planned times of prayer for healing and laying-on-of-hands. Thank God that we are able to be transformed. Turning to the Christ calls for both love and knowledge—a rebirth and radical change of outlook.

4. *Health Promoter Training* and various other educational activities are also key components in the renewal of the mind through knowledge and study. St. Luke's has written and tested a two-part curriculum to train volunteers as promoters of health. Each of the sessions of the two units synthesizes and integrates scripture, spiritual disciplines, and general world view and wholeness concepts with psychosocial, clinical, and health-care skills. The Health Promoter is also given exposure to basic human anatomy, physiology, and common disease processes. Health promoters are taught to consider individuals in their social, economic, and ecological context. We challenge people to grow by providing opportunities that not only stimu-

late their interest but also lead to transformation in their own values, attitudes, and life-styles. It is one thing to talk about spiritual renewal and growth; it is another thing to experience it. We can *believe* in the Risen Christ, but until we *know* him, he remains for the most part in our head and not in our heart.

I would like to share the scripture meditation from the Health Promoter Training session entitled *Integration/Depression*. It can help us to learn to care for the whole person.

"Out of the depths I cry to you, O Lord; Lord, hear my voice!" (Ps 130:1). Psalm 130, like many of the psalms, expresses the anguish of someone caught in the gloom of depression and despair. Some of us may never have known the "depths" of despair, but surely all of us at times have felt "weighed down," "depressed," maybe even "crushed in spirit." From these depths we may indeed cry, but most often we feel powerless to lift ourselves out. What do we do? To whom can we turn?

Again it is important to remember that we do not go to Scripture to find answers to our questions. Rather, we find in Scripture an approach, a connection with people who have lived as we live, suffered as we suffer, rejoiced as we rejoice. We find that ours is not an isolated feeling; we find that we are not alone. Scripture is full of people who have known depression and despair. We will look at one—Job.

Job, as you may recall, was a renowned, successful businessman. He had a good family, many social friends, and was a well-respected member of the community. And then tragedy struck: his cattle and camels were stolen and his herdsmen killed; lightning struck and killed his sheep and shepherds, and a windstorm destroyed his home. Then his own body turned against him, and he broke out in boils from ". . . the soles of his feet to the crown of his head." He seemed cursed.

Let's look at that scenario in our own lives: tragedy strikes from the outside; we lose treasured possessions, but with them often goes our sense of accomplishment and success, our pride and sense of self. Then our bodies, which hold all this stress, begin to show the wear. We become "wasted." In Job's words: "My spirit is broken. . . . I am indeed mocked, and as their provocation mounts, my eyes grow dim. . . . my eye has grown blind with anguish, and all my frame is shrunken to a shadow." (Job 17:1, 2, 7).

Crushed and broken in spirit, we feel isolated, rejected, even abhorred. Listen again to Job: "My brethren have withdrawn from me, and my friends are wholly estranged. My kinsfolk and companions neglect me. . . . My breath is abhorred by my wife; I am loathsome to the men of my family. The young children, too, despise me; when I appear, they speak against me. All my intimate friends hold me in horror; those whom I loved have turned against me! My bones cleave to my skin, and I have escaped with my flesh between my teeth" (Job 19:13–20).

A man crushed by tragedy, withered in body, broken in spirit! What can be done for him? What can we as family, friend or Health Promoter do for another? Job's so-called friends give us examples of what *not* to do. Their advice, their "windy words" as Job calls it, cannot penetrate his gloom, cannot touch his heart. To their advice he answers: "I have heard this sort of thing many times; wearisome comforters are you all! Is there no end to windy words?" (Job 16:2–3).

The first gift we can offer is that of *loving presence*. It is not what we say or do, not our advice or answers that are important, but rather our gentle, faithful being with one another. Job does not dismiss the presence of his friends, only their "vain reminders." In fact, he pleads with them: "Pay careful heed to my speech, and give my statement a hearing" (Job 13:17).

Attentive listening to another is a second gift that we can offer. Sometimes that attentive listening will open a safe, receptive space where the other can touch and share what is troubling. That is what Job asks for when he pleads: ". . . call me, and I will respond; or let me speak first and answer me" (Job 13:22).

Listening to another, helping the other to listen to him or herself is so very important. *Journaling* is a way in which you can help yourself or another listen to the whole of your life's experiences.

Another valuable aid is *positive affirmation*. Listen to Job once again: "But as for me, I know that my Vindicator lives, and that he will at last stand forth upon the dust; whom I myself shall see: my own eyes, not another's, shall behold him, and from my flesh, I shall see God . . ." (Job 19:25–26). This kind of positive affirmation lifts Job out of the depths of despair. When all else has failed, his ability to affirm his trust in a loving God sees him through. Even though he knows himself as "blind," he affirms that he shall see. Even though he knows his body as wasted, he affirms that "from my flesh I shall see God." This is the kind of positive affirmation that takes deep root in the body and slowly, gently can lift one out of despair.

Loving presence and attentive listening are gifts that we can offer another. Journaling, as a way of remembering and connecting, and positive affirmations are aids that we can use. Together they can create the fertile soil in which inner healing can take place.[9]

Mental depression is discussed next in the session. Included in the discussion are the major signs and symptoms observable by the individual who is depressed, by his or her family and friends, as well as by someone such as a Health Promoter. The role of the Health Promoter is explored. The most important caring that the Health Promoter can give to a depressed person is: (1) to listen carefully so that he or she might determine some area of hope for the individual, (2) to look for a possible source of hate or anger that is being denied by the person, (3) to explore with the individual ways to release this anger or hate that are not harmful to the individual or others, and (4) to help move the person toward forgiveness in an awareness of God's love and forgiveness through his or her *visible* love and forgiveness.

Traditional and "whole-person" treatment modalities, including counseling and drug therapy, are then introduced and discussed. Prevention is emphasized and is intimately connected to world-view concepts that the Health Promoter can begin to integrate into the person's life patterns. The session concludes with a discussion of positive affirmations and inner healing.

The Health Promoter Training most fully enfleshes the St. Luke experience. But seminars, conferences, workshops, retreats, and various speaking engagements also give us opportunities to share our vision and insights in congregational, educational, and health care settings.

5. *The St. Luke Life Center* affirms that God is the author, renewer, and sustainer of all life and the ultimate source of all healing. Its mission as an integral part of St. Luke Health Ministries is to witness to the healing presence of Jesus Christ and the gospel message and to facilitate the renewal of healing within the church. The Life Center is a dream in the process of becoming as the Spirit moves and guides. In Habbakuk 2:2–3 we are reminded to "write down the vision . . . so that one can read it readily. If it delays, wait for it, it will surely come; it will not be late."

In the early spring of 1982, two women came forth within two weeks of each other and offered their respective farms as a site for the envisioned renewal/retreat healing center. I had written previously about such a place in our newsletter, "In Touch." I had held up the vision before the Lord in prayer for many years and had in fact visualized what it would look like—beautiful rolling hills with woods and a river in a rural area, but readily accessible to the city. In fact, I asked God very specifically. It was my heart's deepest desire; I "craved" it. William James once said, "Any idea constantly held before the mind *must* come into existence." Well, I think the Lord must have a good sense of humor—not just one, but *two* farms!

After a long and careful process of discernment by a task force, we accepted a gift of 130 acres in the scenic Western Run Valley, thirty-five minutes north of downtown Baltimore, Maryland. God be praised for his gentleness with us during the year of negotiations and decision-making. It was difficult for me to yield my individual vision and guidance to corporate discernment. But together we came to the knowledge of the direct, active, immediate leading of the Spirit. Jesus teaches us, "If two of you agree on earth about anything they ask, it will be done for them by my Father in heaven. For where two or three are gathered in my name, there am I in the midst of them" (Mt 18:19–20). Gathered in his name and discerning his will, we could act in unity and with authority.

Through the Life Center, we seek, as wounded people of God ourselves, to respond more fully to Jesus' call to preach, teach, and heal. We have chosen to share life as a community, both resident and nonresident, to create a new environment of love and hope that is nourished by the Spirit. Seeing ourselves as agents of change steeped in prayer, we are attempting to be faithful to the prophetic mission of the healing ministry—to wholeness and justice.

Community members represent a broad spectrum of faith traditions but are all called by the Spirit to witness to the reconciliation possible within the Body of Christ, the church catholic. It is indeed scandalous that Christians remain divided, more often because of issues of power and control than any significant doctrinal differences. Like the Taizé Communities, we hope to witness effectively to the wider body of believers. As an intentional ecumenical community, our commitment is to loving, caring service in the spirit of the compassionate Jesus.

The Life Center is open to anyone who seeks healing and wishes to deepen his or her relationship with God, self, family, and creation. The doors are always open to the powerless, the unloved, the unforgiven. We feel, however, a special burden to minister specifically and directly to the ministers—pastors, religious men and women, and others engaged in full-time ministry. They need time away to let down the barriers, to be themselves, to share their hurts, reflect on their vocation, and then to find healing in prayer, solitude, and loving acceptance. We would also offer renewal of spirit, body, and mind to those hurting persons in other helping and healing professions, such as physicians, nurses, and counselors. By sharing *our* wounds we open up a space that is nonthreatening where others can question and explore without fear of censure. Unless persons in positions of leadership and authority within the church are cared for, those who follow surely will begin to lose heart.

We pray and worship together regularly. Study, quiet time, and creativity in the arts are encouraged—not only for personal joy and satisfaction but also to enhance the life of the community.

Care of the body by proper physical conditioning and nutrition, like prayer, is therapeutic as well as preventive and health promoting. The chapel is a place set aside for worship of God with heart, mind, and soul. The fitness center will be the place set aside for caring for the body.

All living space is being planned to reflect the true meaning of the Life Center, wherein the space itself expresses healing—a whole—in keeping with the natural harmony of the land. Buildings are to be aesthetically balanced and coordinated in shape, color, and overall layout, as well as functional and energy efficient by renewable resources of sun and wind. We feel ourselves responsible to care for the earth and all God's creation.

The retreats have become important times for helping others to open themselves to the Divine Lover, the one who forgives and transforms—the Healer. They are a powerful means to equip the saints for radical discipleship. An integrated and healing inward journey results in an awakened and renewed outward journey. Peace through the cross experienced inwardly leads to taking up one's cross for the sake of peace and justice outwardly. After a meaningful retreat on healing and the spiritual disciplines, we received a beautiful letter from a seminary student:

> Today I decided to write down my reflections on the weekend we experienced together. I wanted to share those with you, so that you might be affirmed in the job you did as leaders. That's what the whole weekend was for me—an affirmation of who I am and what I am about . . . Friday night during the Grand Silence I felt directed to turn to Hebrews 10, and there were several verses that I hadn't noticed before, but which expressed what I needed and had come seeking.
>
> > Let us draw near with a true heart in full assurance of faith. Let us hold fast the confession of our hope, without wavering, for he who promised is faithful; and let us consider how to stir up one another to love and good works, not neglecting to meet together . . . but encouraging one another. . . . But recall the former days when, after you were enlightened, you endured a hard struggle with sufferings . . . Therefore, do not throw away your

confidence, which has a great reward. For you have need of endurance, so that you may do the will of God and receive what is promised. . . . But we are not of those who shrink back and are destroyed, but of those who have faith and keep their souls. (Heb 10:22–25, 32, 35–36, 39)

I shared at lunch the notion that the "spirit of weakness" the Spirit spoke to me about during the reflection time after the Bible study was my problem of low self-esteem. And there it all was in those verses: assurance, hope without wavering, stir up and encourage one another—all the things I've lacked because too often I had thrown away my confidence, shrank back, given up to discouragement and depression . . . not using my faith.

. . . How could I minister to, encourage, and stir up others to good works when I myself got so discouraged? It was as if Jesus, in that time of silence, was reassuring me that he was healing me and that I was in the process of becoming the "daughter of Abraham" made whole.

The Lord forms each of us as the potter molds the clay; we are the work of his hand. But often we do not like our handle or the shape of our fragile vessel. We may feel misshapen, unappealing, unusable. I sometimes question the worth of my very personhood, not even considering the ministry of health and healing to which I am called. How can I care for the whole person when I myself feel so out of touch and inappropriate? I sometimes question, if not reject outright, the Potter's handiwork. Can anything good come forth from such a broken vessel? And yet the call to wholeness for me, and for each person, is to recognize and to hold within that precious treasure that is life itself—Jesus, the Christ. It is to choose life.

Our society is often seductive in its call to self-fulfillment, self-esteem, self-enhancement in an attempt to experience a full, healthy life. Yet Jesus clearly states that, "For whoever would save his life will lose it; and whoever loses his life for my sake, he will save it" (Lk 9:24). The paradox, then, in choosing life and in seeking healing is to die to self. The seed of grain falls into the ground and dies in order to become wheat. So, too, the pain and brokenness of my humanity must be transformed, so that I can become whole and proclaim with the Apostle Paul, "It is no longer I who live, but Christ who lives in me" (Gal 2:20). The words of the prophet Jeremiah ring true, "You have seduced me, Yahweh, and I have let myself be seduced. You have overpowered me: you were the stronger" (Jer 20:7, JB). Thanks be to God for his great love and mercy!

Epilogue

We have come full circle from the theoretical and cognitive to the practical and pragmatic—from neutral living and death to growth and transformation. Challenged by fear with disease, disintegration, and premature death, our Lord invites us into the way of love, justice, and peace—to move in awareness toward integration, toward health and wholeness. We are not victims; we are given glimpses of a new reality and the opportunity to respond, not only for ourselves but in service to others.

The gospel message is not neutral; it requires a radical response. We are called to choose health and life, full and abundant, a life of discipleship. To be healed is to be transformed. To be healed is to dare to risk change as an individual and as a society. To be healed is to move beyond pious utterings to a real encounter with the Risen Christ. Healing sets us free to be the people of God in a broken world.

As Christians, we can really know and experience Jesus' presence and power; we can turn the world upside down for the sake of the kingdom. May our mission and ministry of healing and reconciliation flow out of obedience to the crucified and Risen Lord. Prepared and expecting to forgive, love, and serve, we proclaim that the kingdom is in and among us now and forever. Alleluia! Amen.

Notes

Chapter 1 / Living in Neutral

1. Frederick Franck, *The Zen of Seeing* (New York: Vintage Books, 1973), p. 4.

2. Stuart J. Kingma, M.D., "A Unified View of Healing—the Centrality of Hope and Reconciliation," Study paper, p. 2. Dr. Kingma is the former director of the Christian Medical Commission, World Council of Churches, Geneva, Switzerland.

3. Leighton Cluff, M.D., Vice President, The Robert Wood Johnson Foundation. Cited in his keynote address at the Lutheran Church in America Conference on "Health, Healing, and Health Care." Omaha, Nebraska, May 13-15, 1983.

4. U.S. Department of Health and Human Services, Public Health Service. *Health: United States, 1981.* Hyattsville, MD: U.S. Government Printing Office, 1981.

5. Regina Sara Ryan and John W. Travis, M.D. *Wellness Workbook* (Berkeley, California: Ten Speed Press, 1981), p. 4. This is a marvelous book for exploring the meaning of health and wellness.

6. The fight or flight response was first described by Walter Cannon in 1914. This response enables a person to react to a stress factor by mobilizing all of his/her resources so that he/she may either fight or run. This may include the following physiological responses: The heart increases its pumping activity and rate. The major muscles of the body "tense." There is sweating of the palms and soles and increased visual perception. The breathing rate increases and food digestion shuts down. When any of these becomes chronic, illness may occur. For an excellent discussion of the fight or flight response, read *Stress for Success* by Morse and Furst.

7. Kenneth R. Pelletier, *Mind as Healer, Mind as Slayer* (New York: Dell Publishing Co., 1977), pp. 69, 70.

8. Claudia Wallis, "Stress: Can We Cope?" *Time*, June 6, 1983, p. 50.

9. Fritjof Capra, *The Turning Point: Science, Society, and the Rising Culture* (Toronto: Bantam Books, 1982), p. 247. An excellent book on the reconciliation of science and the human spirit.

10. Jim Wallis, *The Call to Conversion: Recovering the Gospel for These Times* (San Francisco: Harper and Row, 1981), p. 48. This is an outstanding pastoral from a contemporary prophetic voice.

Chapter 2 / Disease, Disintegration, and Death

1. I am indebted to my friend, Dr. John Travis, whose *Illness/Wellness Continuum* is the foundation for this model. See the Ryan and Travis *Wellness Workbook* cited above. Further elaboration and clarity came from my friend, Elaine McCarthy, and others, to whom this model was presented in numerous seminars and conferences.

2. "Cartesian" refers to the seventeenth-century philosophy of René Descartes, who is usually regarded as the founder of modern philosophy. He held a firm belief in the certainty of scientific knowledge, which lies at the very basis of Cartesian philosophy and the world view derived from it. Cartesian certainty is mathematical in its essential nature.

3. Fritjof Capra, *The Turning Point*, pp. 145, 146.

4. James Nelson, *Embodiment* (Minneapolis: Augsburg, 1978), p. 30.

5. Ibid., p. 32.

6. Ibid., p. 33.

7. Ibid., p. 77.

8. I had learned to pray through my acquaintance with Agnes Sanford. See the numerous books written by Agnes Sanford.

9. Richard Foster, *Freedom of Simplicity* (San Francisco: Harper and Row, 1981). Foster is original, clear, and concise. See especially chapters 5 and 6.

10. Stuart J. Kingma, M.D., "A Unified View of Healing—the Centrality of Hope and Reconciliation," p.6.

11. Leo E. Missinne, W.F., Ph.D., "The Problem of Loneliness," *Human Development*, 4, no. 2, Summer 1983, p. 9.

Chapter 3 / *Living in Awareness*

1. Fritjof Capra, *The Turning Point*, pp. 25, 26.
2. Ibid., pp. 47, 48.
3. John Risley, "Liberation Spirituality," *Spirituality Today*, Summer 1983, 35, no. 2, p. 128.
4. Morton Kelsey, *Encounter with God* (Minneapolis: Bethany Fellowship, 1972), p. 151.
5. Ibid., pp. 137, 138.
6. Capra, *The Turning Point*, p. 91.
7. Ibid., p. 87.
8. Ibid., p. 91.
9. Ibid., p. 123.
10. Reprinted from Morton Kelsey, *The Other Side of Silence* (New York: Paulist Press, 1976), p. 37. Kelsey first developed this model in his book *Encounter with God*. It is a basic paradigm for his writings.
11. Morton Kelsey, *Encounter with God*, pp. 154, 155.
12. Paul Tillich, *The New Being* (New York: Charles Scribner's Sons, 1955), p. 23.
13. Paul Tillich, *Systematic Theology* (New York: Harper and Row, 1967), p. 166.
14. Morton Kelsey, *Healing and Christianity* (New York: Harper and Row, 1973), p. 67. This book is the first comprehensive history of sacramental healing in the Christian Church from biblical times to the present. It took Professor Kelsey approximately twenty years to compile the material for it.

Chapter 4 / *Transformation, Integration, and Growth*

1. Richard Foster, *Richard J. Foster's Study Guide for Celebration of Discipline* (San Francisco: Harper and Row, 1983), p. 6.
2. Walter Wink, *The Bible in Human Transformation* (Philadelphia: Fortress Press, 1973), pp. 78, 79. The poem is from T.S. Eliot, "East Coker" in *Four Quartets* (New York: Harcourt, Brace and Company, 1943), p. 15.
3. Keith Clark, *Make Space, Make Symbols: A Personal Journey into Prayer.* (Notre Dame, Indiana: Ave Maria Press, 1979).
4. Jim Wallis, *The Call to Conversion*, pp. 6, 7.
5. Abraham Maslow, *Toward a Psychology of Being* (New York: D. Van Nostrand Company, 1968), p. 46.
6. Donald P. McNeill, Douglas A. Morrison, and Henri J. M. Nouwen, *Compassion: A Reflection on the Christian Life* (Garden City: Doubleday and Co., Inc., 1982), p. 96.
7. James S. Gordon, M.D. and Doris B. Haire, "Alternatives in

Childbirth," Health for the Whole Person, Hastings, Fadiman and Gordon, eds. (Toronto: Bantam Books, 1980), pp. 311–342.

8. Morton Kelsey, Healing and Christianity, p. 301

Chapter 5 / Living in Wholeness

1. Richard Foster, Celebration of Discipline: The Path to Spiritual Growth (San Francisco: Harper and Row, 1978), p. 30.

2. Ibid., p. 30.

3. David C. Jacobsen, Clarity in Prayer, Prayer Renewal Workshops, 1979, p. 25.

4. Ibid., p. 28.

5. McNeill, Morrison, and Nouwen, Compassion, p. 36.

6. Agnes Sanford, The Healing Light (St. Paul, Minnesota: Macalester Park Publishing Co., 1947). This classic was Agnes Sanford's first book; the manuscript sat in a drawer for many years before it was published. In later years, Mrs. Sanford was asked by many scientists how she knew about light and energy before they had even proposed their theories of quantum mechanics. She replied, "He told me!"

7. Hal Hellman, "Guiding Light," Psychology Today, April 1982, pp. 22–28. Philip C. Hughes, "The Use of Light and Color in Health," in Health for the Whole Person, pp. 294–308. This particular chapter, as well as each chapter of the book, has an excellent list of references and an annotated bibliography.

8. Fritjof Capra, The Turning Point, p. 88.

9. Vladimir Lossky, The Mystical Theology of the Eastern Church (London: James Clarke and Co., Ltd., 1957), p. 218. First published in Paris in 1944 under the title Essai sur la Théologie Mystique de l'Eglise d'Orient. It was translated by a small group of members of the Fellowship of St. Alban and St. Serguis, an unofficial body that exists to promote understanding between Eastern and Western Christians. Chapter Eleven, "The Divine Light," is powerful and very important.

10. Ibid., p. 220.

11. Ibid., p. 223.

12. Ibid., p. 223.

13. Ibid., p. 224.

14. The New Age of Healing (Los Angeles: Science of Mind Publications, 1979), pp. 34–49.

15. Capra, The Turning Point, p. 89.

16. Paul Tillich, The New Being, p. 38.

17. Foster, Celebration of Discipline, p. 127.

18. Bernard Grad, "Some Biological Effects of the 'Laying On of Hands': A Review of Experiments with Animals and Plants," Journal

of the American Society for Physical Research, 59, no. 2, April 1965, pp. 95–126.

Dolores Krieger, "Therapeutic Touch: The Imprimatur of Nursing," *American Journal of Nursing,* 75, May 1975, pp. 784–787.

19. Jim Wallis, *The Call to Conversion,* p. 12.

20. Ibid., p. 109.

21. "Easter people" refers to persons who, in their Christian faith, believe in and live out of the centrality of the resurrection of Jesus Christ. The Christ who was crucified and died also defeated Death and was raised from the dead. He is risen and lives eternally. He can be encountered in our experience now, and offers us the way to salvation— health and wholeness.

Chapter 6 / Caring for the Whole Person

1. Ralph E. Peterson, *A Study of the Healing Church and Its Ministry: The Health Care Apostolate* (New York: The Lutheran Church in America, 1982), p. 9.

2. Morton Kelsey, *Healing and Christianity,* p. 223.

3. Fritjof Capra, *The Turning Point,* pp. 123, 124.

4. Ibid., p. 43.

5. Gordon Dalbey, "Recovering Healing Prayer," *The Christian Century,* June 9–16, 1982, pp. 690–693.

6. James Gordon, "The Paradigm of Holistic Medicine," *Health for the Whole Person,* p. 17.

7. Jim Wallis, *Agenda for Biblical People* (New York: Harper and Row, 1976), p. 95.

8. Morton Kelsey, *Encounter with God,* p. 173.

9. My friend and colleague Frances Cavey, SUSC, is a gifted writer, as well as pastoral counselor and educator. Fran lives and expresses an intimate relationship with the Lord and is a cherished member of the St. Luke Health Ministries staff and community.

Bibliography

BONHOEFFER, DIETRICH
1959   *The Cost of Discipleship*. New York: The Macmillan Company.
1954   *Life Together*. New York: Harper and Row, Publishers.

CAPRA, FRITJOF
1982   *The Turning Point*. Toronto: Bantam Books.
1975   *The Tao of Physics*. Berkeley, Calif. Shambhala.

COUSINS, NORMAN
1979   *Anatomy of an Illness*. New York: W. W. Norton.

ELLUL, JACQUES
1948   *The Presence of the Kingdom*. New York: The Seabury Press.

FOSTER, RICHARD J.
1981   *Freedom of Simplicity*. New York: Harper and Row, Publishers.
1978   *Celebration of Discipline*. New York: Harper and Row, Publishers.

FOX, MATTHEW
1979   *A Spirituality Named Compassion and the Healing of the Global Village, Humpty Dumpty and Us*. Minneapolis: Winston Press.
1983   *Original Blessing*. Santa Fe: Bear & Company, Inc.

FRANK, JEROME D.
1969   *Persuasion and Healing*. New York: Schocken Books.

FROST, EVELYN
1940   *Christian Healing: A Considerationn of the Place of Spiritual Healing in the Church Today in the Light of the Doctrine and Practice of the Ante-Nicene Church*. London: A. R. Mowbray and Company.

114

GUTIERREZ, GUSTAVO
 1973   *A Theology of Liberation.* Maryknoll, N. Y.: Orbis Books.
HEISENBURG, WERNER
 1962   *Physics and Philosophy.* New York: Harper and Row, Publishers.
HOFFMAN, BENGT
 1976   *Luther and the Mystics.* Minneapolis: Augsburg Publishing House.
ILLICH, IVAN
 1976   *Medical Nemesis.* New York: Pantheon Books.
KELSEY, MORTON T.
 1982   *Christo-Psychology.* New York: Crossroad.
 1976   *The Other Side of Silence: A Guide to Christian Meditation.* New York: Paulist Press.
 1973   *Healing and Christianity.* New York: Harper and Row, Publishers.
 1972   *Encounter With God.* Minneapolis: Bethany Fellowship, Inc.
KUHN, THOMAS S.
 1970   *The Structure of Scientific Revolutions.* Chicago: University of Chicago Press.
LARSON, BRUCE
 1978   *The Meaning and Mystery of Being Human.* Waco, Tex.: Word Books.
MACNUTT, FRANCIS
 1977   *The Power to Heal.* Notre Dame: Ave Maria Press.
 1974   *Healing.* Notre Dame: Ave Maria Press.
MADDOCKS, MORRIS
 1981   *The Christian Healing Ministry.* London: SPCK.
MAY, GERALD G.
 1982   *Care of Mind/Care of Spirit.* New York: Harper and Row, Publishers.
MCNEILL, DONALD P., DOUGLAS A. MORRISON, AND HENRI J. M. NOUWEN
 1982   *Compassion: A Reflection on the Christian Life.* Garden City, N. Y.: Doubleday and Company, Inc.

NOUWEN, HENRI J. M.
1972   *The Wounded Healer*. Garden City, N. Y.: Double-day and Company, Inc.

PELLETIER, KENNETH R.
1977   *Mind as Healer, Mind as Slayer*. New York: Dell Publishing Company.

PETERMAN, MARY E.
1974   *Healing, A Spiritual Adventure*. Philadelphia: Fortress Press.

PETERSON, RALPH E.
1982   *A Study of the Healing Church and Its Ministry*. New York: The Lutheran Church in America.

RYAN, REGINA SARA, AND JOHN W. TRAVIS.
1981   *Wellness Workbook*. Berkeley, Calif.: Ten Speed Press.

SANFORD, AGNES
1969   *The Healing Power of the Bible*. Philadelphia: Trumpet Books, published by A. J. Homan Company.
1966   *The Healing Gifts of the Spirit*. Philadelphia: Trumpet Books, published by A. J. Homan Company.
1958   *Behold Your God*. St. Paul: Macalester Park Publishing Company.
1947   *The Healing Light*. St. Paul: Macalester Park Publishing Company.

SCANLAN, MICHAEL
1974   *Inner Healing*. New York: Paulist Press.

SCHELL, JONATHAN
1982   *The Fate of the Earth*. New York: Knopf.

SCHUMACHER, E. F.
1973   *Small Is Beautiful: Economics as if People Mattered*. New York: Harper and Row, Publishers.

SELYE, HANS
1974   *Stress Without Distress*. New York: J. B. Lippincott Company.

SIDER, RONALD J.
1977   *Rich Christians in an Age of Hunger: A Biblical Study*. Downers Grove, Ill.: Inter-Varsity Press.

SIMONTON, O. CARL, STEPHANIE MATTHEWS-SIMONTON, AND JAMES
CREIGHTON
1978   *Getting Well Again.* Los Angeles: Tarcher.
SOJOURNERS, ED.
1981   A Matter of Faith: A Study Guide for Churches on
the Nuclear Arms Race. Washington, D. C.: Sojourners.
STRINGFELLOW, WILLIAM
1973   *An Ethic for Christians and Other Aliens in a
Strange Land.* Waco, Tex.: Word Books, Publishers.
TAMEZ, ELSA
1982   *Bible of the Oppressed.* Maryknoll, N. Y.: Orbis
Books.
TOURNIER, PAUL
1964   *The Whole Person in a Broken World.* New York:
Harper and Row, Publishers.
1957   *The Meaning of Persons.* New York: Harper and
Row, Publishers.
VANIER, JEAN
1979   *Community and Growth.* New York: Paulist Press.
WALLIS, JIM
1981   *Call to Conversion.* New York: Harper and Row,
Publishers.
1976   *Agenda for Biblical People.* New York: Harper and
Row, Publishers.
WINK, WALTER
1980   *Transforming Bible Study.* Nashville: Abingdon.
1973   *The Bible in Human Transformation.* Philadelphia:
Fortress Press.
ZUKAV, GARY.
1979   *The Dancing Wu Li Masters.* Toronto: Bantam
Books.